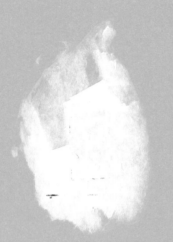

THE
HERBAL
REMEDY
HANDBOOK

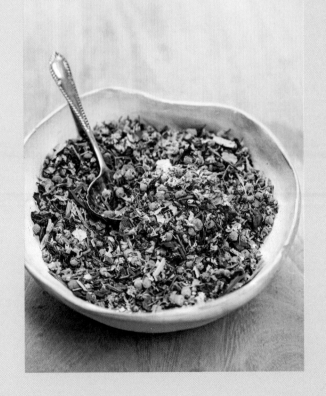

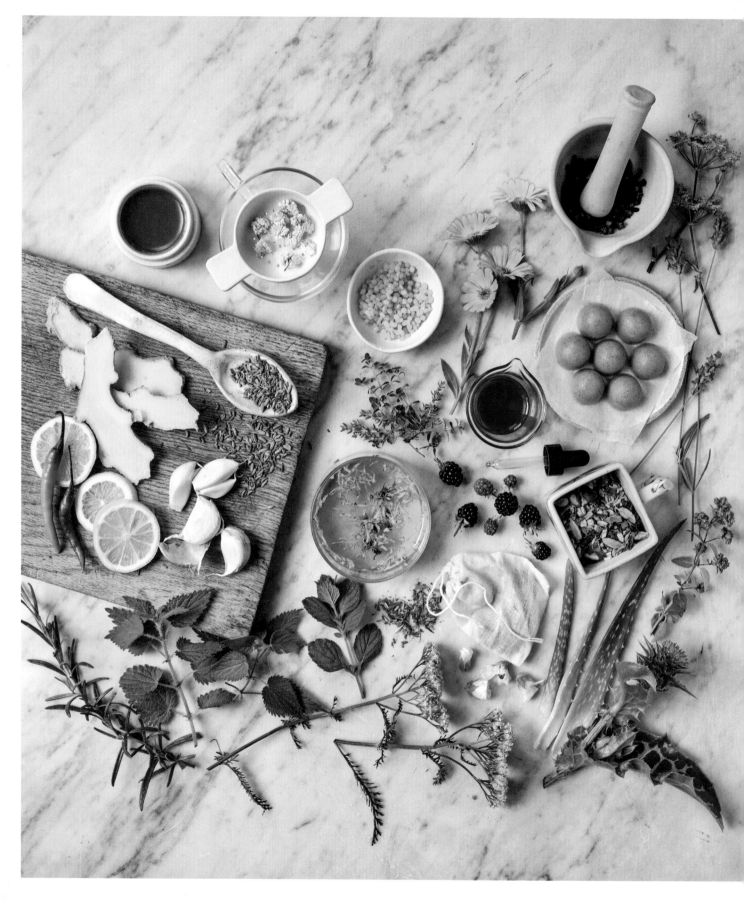

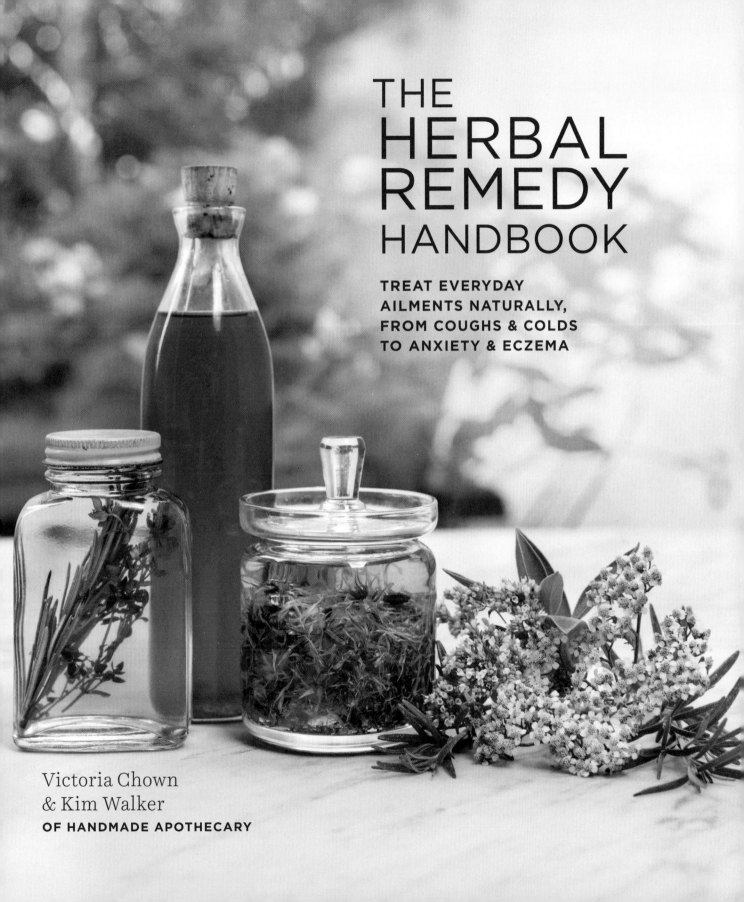

THE HERBAL REMEDY HANDBOOK

**TREAT EVERYDAY
AILMENTS NATURALLY,
FROM COUGHS & COLDS
TO ANXIETY & ECZEMA**

Victoria Chown
& Kim Walker
OF HANDMADE APOTHECARY

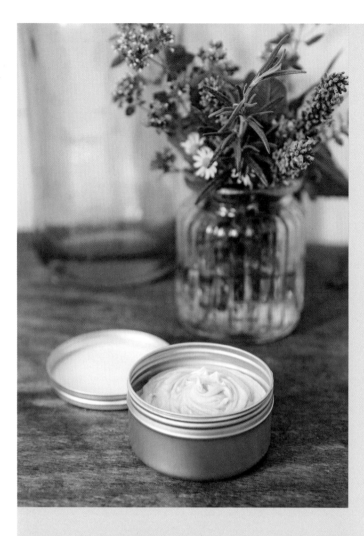

Photographer Sarah Cuttle
Design Ketchup
Props stylist Ali Allen
Project Editor Sophie Allen
Editorial Assistant Sarah Kyle
Production Lisa Pinnell

Disclaimer: The authors and publishers do not accept any responsibility for loss, harm or damage from the use or misuse of this book, or your failure to seek proper medical advice.

An Hachette UK Company
www.hachette.co.uk

First published in Great Britain in 2019 by
Kyle Books, an imprint of Kyle Cathie Ltd
Carmelite House
50 Victoria Embankment
London EC4Y 0DZ
www.kylebooks.co.uk

Distributed in the US by Hachette Book Group,
1290 Avenue of the Americas, 4th and 5th Floors,
New York, NY 10104.

Distributed in Canada by Canadian Manda Group,
664 Annette St., Toronto, Ontario, Canada M6S 2C8.

ISBN: 978 085783 502 4

10 9 8 7 6 5 4 3 2 1

A Cataloguing in Publication record for this title is available from the British Library.

Printed and bound in China

CONTENTS

INTRODUCTION

There's nothing like the feeling of making your own remedies. Whether it is the creative bliss of standing over a bubbling pot of herbal syrup, or simply the feeling of knowing exactly what to reach for to soothe a sore throat, a little herbal knowledge, wisely used, is a hugely self-empowering act. In the West until the 20th century, few people would have been able to afford access to formal healthcare, and so relied on knowledge passed down to them, or on a local herbalist to have remedies to ease their pains. Much of this herbal knowledge has faded, or been sidelined as 'old-wives' tales' but, like weeds, the knowledge won't just disappear and is bound to keep popping up when you least expect it.

Our last book, *The Handmade Apothecary*, focused on foraging outdoors for herbs to create your own herbal medicines. In this book, however, we have shared some simple, tried-and-tested remedies and recipes that use kitchen cupboard staples, can be 'foraged' from the local supermarket or products that are commonly found in health food shops or herbal suppliers. We have had lots of fun concocting and creating herbal remedies for this book and we hope that you enjoy rediscovering the art of making your own medicines, too.

HOW TO USE THIS BOOK

This book is intended as a reference guide to some traditional and common herbal remedies, enabling you to treat minor ailments and illnesses at home. It provides recipes for basic herbal preparations (pages 12–27), which can be tailored to individual needs using the recommended traditionally used herbs listed in each ailment section.

Herbal medicine is a holistic practice, meaning that it aims to understand the cause(s) of an illness rather than just treat the symptoms. A holistic approach to health is especially important where illness is chronic, severe or has very complicated origins; in these cases it is always advisable to seek advice from a medical herbalist before using herbs medicinally at home: see the 'Finding a herbalist' section on page 172. We also encourage you to explore the holistic herbal approach and discover more about herbs, and a list of recommended books can be found in 'A herbalist's library' on page 173.

The recipes in this book use ingredients commonly found in hedgerows, supermarkets, online and from herbalists and herbal suppliers: see the 'Sourcing herbs' (page 10) and 'Suppliers of herbs and ingredients' (page 172) sections. Throughout the book we have used the common names of the herbs, but it is important to know the scientific names (e.g. elderflower: *Sambucus nigra*) to ensure you have the correct medicinal plant, as sometimes different plants can share the same common name but have different uses. These can be found in the Latin glossary on page 170.

Overall, this book will provide guidance on making simple herbal preparations at home, allowing you to incorporate herbal medicines into your life for healthy, empowering self-care.

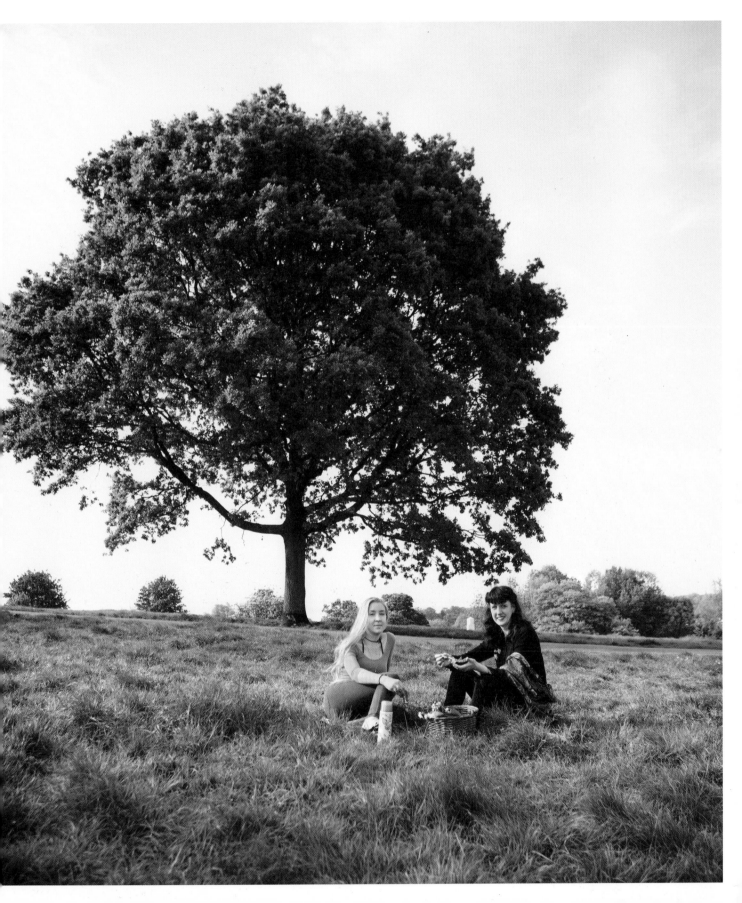

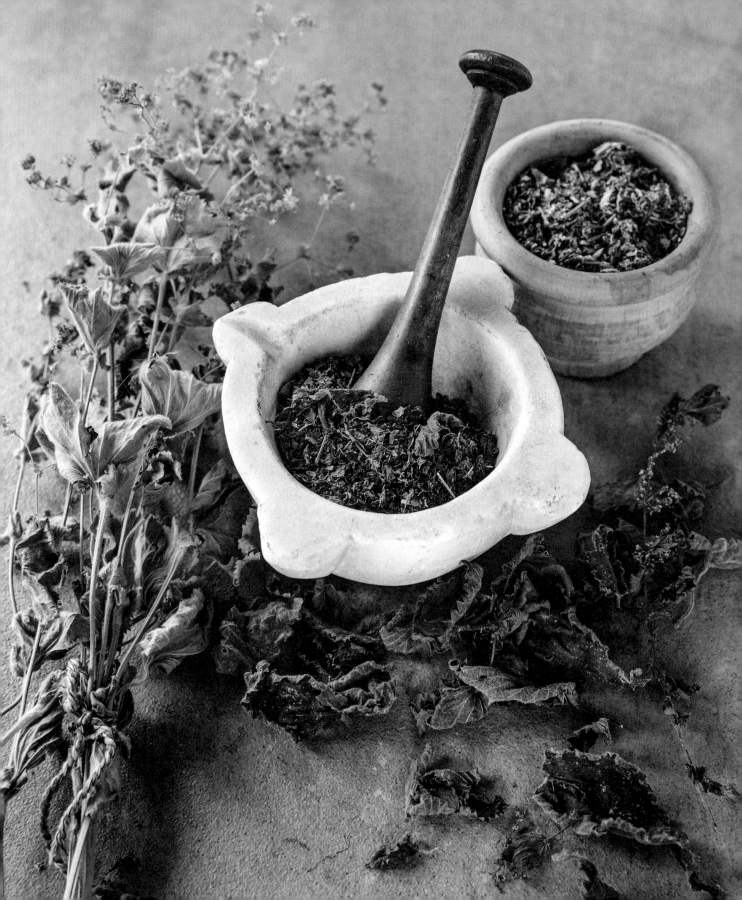

HOW TO USE HERBS SAFELY

Herbal medicine is the oldest form of medicine. The herbs chosen for this book have a long traditional use and have stood the test of time, and some have emerging scientific research supporting their efficacy. When used correctly, herbs can offer a safe and natural form of medicine for a wide range of illnesses, acting as a preventative and to enhance general wellbeing. Although herbal medicine is a 'natural' form of healing, it must not be confused with being entirely harmless and appropriate and sensible care is needed when using them. Herbs have great therapeutic value; their chemical constituents have the ability to interact with and affect the cells, tissues, organs and systems of the body. They must be treated with respect and used with some caution. This is especially true for pregnant women, the very young, the very old, those who suffer from chronic or severe illness and those on medication. If in doubt, see a herbalist before embarking on a herbal healing journey.

DOSAGE

Like prescription drugs, herbs have certain doses that must be adhered to for effective and safe use. Unless otherwise instructed, the standard dosage for herbal treatments are as follows:

INFUSIONS AND DECOCTIONS 2 teaspoons of fresh, or 1 teaspoon of dried herbs to 1 cup of water, 1–2 times daily

TINCTURES AND GLYCERITES 2–5ml (½–1 teaspoon) in a little water, 1–3 times daily

HERBAL INFUSED HONEY 1–2 teaspoons, 1–3 times daily

SYRUPS 10–30ml (2 teaspoons–1 fl oz) on its own, in a cold or warm drink, up to 3 times daily

DISCLAIMER

- The information in this book is for educational purposes, to inform the reader about traditional remedies and approaches in Western herbal medicine. It is not intended for self-diagnosis or as a replacement for professional medical advice and treatment.
- Do not use any remedies on children under the age of two years without first checking with a herbalist.
- Patch-test any external remedies 24 hours before using to check for any reactions or allergies.
- If you have any pre-existing conditions, are trying to conceive, are pregnant or breastfeeding, are on any medication including, but not limited to, the contraceptive pill, painkillers and antidepressants, seek advice from a qualified medical practitioner and herbalist before you try herbal remedies.
- The authors and publishers do not accept any responsibility for loss, harm or damage from the use or misuse of this book, or your failure to seek proper medical advice.

SOURCING HERBS

Sourcing good-quality herbs is an essential part of creating your own remedies. Here is a brief guide to growing, foraging or buying in the best herbs.

GROWING HERBS

Ideally, grow your own herbs if you can – that way you know they are the best quality possible. Even if you don't have a garden, herbs, particularly culinary ones, grow well in pots that can sit on windowsills. Well-established herbs from a garden centre, or from cuttings from friends' plants, will be better than those sold in the supermarket, which tend not to last long. If you don't have a garden, then garden shares, community gardens or allotments are great options for getting involved with growing your own.

FORAGING FOR HERBS

Foraging is a popular way to source local herbs. However, for safety reasons, it is vital to gain the right skills before heading out to gather your own. Correct identification is important to ensure that your herbs are, at the minimum, suitable for the purpose you wish, and most importantly are not poisonous. Buy a good guidebook or two, then find a local plant identification group or walk and test out your skills with an expert. Also check out how to forage legally, sustainably and safely. Ensure you pick from safe areas (free from animal faeces, heavy metal contamination and pollution), and of course protect and preserve precious areas of wildlife. Once you have been initiated into sensible foraging practices, it is a wonderful way to get outside and reconnect with nature – with plants, their histories and uses.

DRYING HERBS

Herbs are seasonal and best harvested in their prime. Drying herbs enables them to be kept for year-round use. Delicate plant parts such as flowers and leaves can be dried by laying them out on a tea towel or piece of muslin, or on a drying rack; or for herbs on long stalks, tie them with a piece of string and hang them up. For thicker plant parts such as sliced roots and berries, lay out the plant material on a baking tray lined with baking parchment and place in an oven on the lowest setting with the door open slightly. Alternatively, use a dehydrator. (Depending on the plant material, this may take up to a few hours. They are ready once the item is completely dry. You can check this by seeing if the stems will snap.)

Flowers, herbs and 'lighter' plant material are at their best stored for up to one year. 'Tougher' material such as seeds, bark and roots can be kept for up to two years. But use your senses – if things no longer smell fresh or herby, are a shadow of their former selves or musty, it is time to discard them. Store herbs in an airtight container in a cool, dark place.

BUYING HERBS AND OTHER INGREDIENTS

As a rule of thumb when buying herbs, choose those that retain a good colour from the original plant and smell fresh and herby, not musty. Dried leafy herbs for culinary use from the supermarket are not always sufficient quality for medicinal use, and are expensive in the amounts required. Spices are usually of a fairly good quality from supermarkets.

Trusted herbal sellers should be sought and will be recognised by their transparency on where the herb was sourced and how they ensure sustainable practice. They should also be able to tell you the scientific name of the herb, to ensure you get the plant you expect. A suggested list of places from which to source herbs can be found on pages 171–2, which also provide sources for basic ingredients such as oils, clays and waxes.

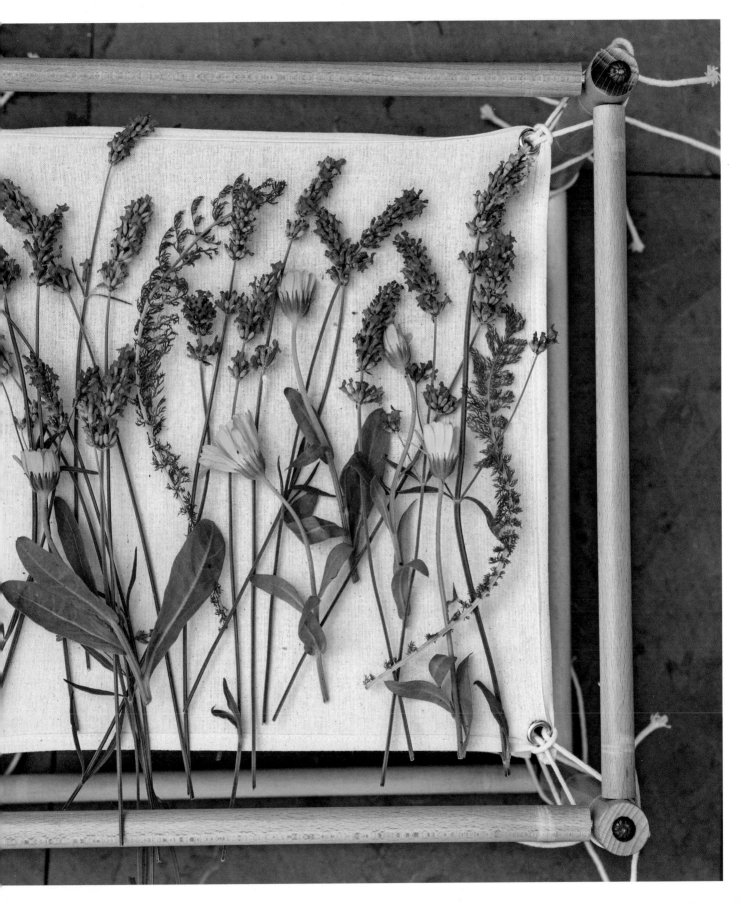

INTERNAL REMEDIES
INFUSIONS & DECOCTIONS

Turning fresh herbs into remedies and preparations is a great way to extract their beneficial properties, preserve them for year-round use and convert them to a form that can be easily used. Internal remedies include infusions, tinctures and honeys; for external remedies, see page 20.

Infusions and decoctions are water-based preparations. Infusions are ideal for the more delicate parts of a herb, such as the leaves and flowers. Tougher plant material like bark, dried berries, mushrooms and roots require more time to extract plant compounds via a process that creates a decoction (see opposite).

Long/overnight infusions

Long/overnight infusions are used to extract heavier molecules, such as minerals from herbs. This method is great for nutritionally dense herbs such as nettle, red clover, oatstraw and horsetail. They also extract astringent tannins very well from, for example, lady's mantle and raspberry leaf. They are made in exactly the same way as a standard infusion, except the herbs are left to steep for 4–12 hours.

Use 1–2 teaspoons of fresh or dried herbs to 1 cup (240ml/9fl oz) of boiling water. Place the plant material in a teapot or lidded vessel, cover with the hot water and a lid, and leave to infuse for 4–12 hours. If leaving this mix to infuse for more than 4 hours, it is advisable to allow it to cool, then keep it in the fridge for the remainder of the infusion period. Strain out and discard the herbs and drink.

Hot infusions

This is similar to making a cup of tea. Hot infusions are great because they are fast. Using boiling water speeds up the breakdown of plant cell walls to release the plant's medicinal effects and allows you to have a remedy ready for use within as little as 10 minutes. Green leafy herbs and flowers are best suited to hot infusions, as are those high in aromatic oils, as the heat helps to extract volatile oil compounds. It is important to use a teapot or a cup with a lid, as volatile oils escape into the air with the steam, condense on the lid and run back down into the infusion, meaning they are in your cup rather than floating away (a saucer on top of a mug will do the trick).

Use 1–2 teaspoons of fresh or dried herbs to 1 cup (240ml/9 fl oz) of boiling water. Place the plant material in a teapot or lidded vessel, cover with the hot water and a lid and leave to infuse for 5–10 minutes. Strain out and discard the herbs and enjoy.

TO USE Drink 1–3 cups a day.

Cold infusions

As the name suggests, cold infusions are made in the absence of heat. So to break down plant cell walls and allow them to release their medicinal chemicals, they need a bit of persuasion in the form of a good bashing. These are best suited to nutrient-rich, leafy green plants, and some flowers, such as cleavers, nettle and oatstraw. Other herbs that are well suited to cold infusions are demulcent herbs, which release their soothing mucilaginous properties (in the form of goo) when left to soak in cold water; these include psyllium husk, slippery elm powder and marshmallow root.

Bash a small handful of your herb of choice in a pestle and mortar or in a strong bowl with the end of a rolling pin, place in a jug and cover with 600ml (20 fl oz) of cold water. Place this in the fridge and leave to infuse overnight or for a minimum of 4 hours. Strain out and discard the plant material and flavour the drink with a slice of lemon, if preferred.

TO USE Drink 1–3 cups a day.

SHELF LIFE Cold infusions can be kept in the fridge for up to 2 days.

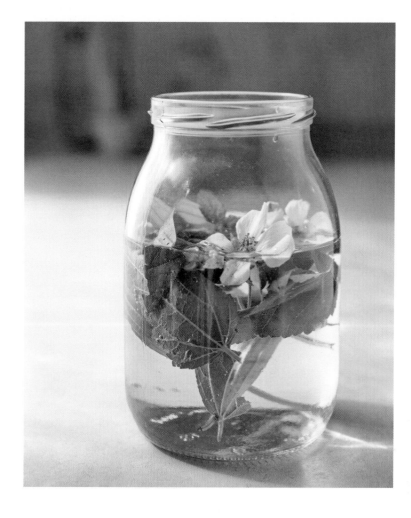

Decoctions

Decoctions are similar to hot infusions, but instead of just steeping the herb in hot water, the plant material is simmered for a while to break down tougher plant cellulose. Decoctions are best suited to berries, seeds, mushrooms, roots and bark.

Place 1–3 teaspoons of fresh or dried plant material in a saucepan, pour over 2 cups (480ml/18 fl oz) of water and cover with a lid. Bring to the boil, then reduce to a gentle simmer for 10–20 minutes. Strain out and discard the plant material and drink.

TO USE Drink 1–3 cups a day.

TINCTURES

A tincture is a hydro-alcoholic extract of a herb: both water and alcohol are used to extract the medicinal qualities of a plant. This allows for both water-soluble and some fat-soluble plant chemicals to be extracted. Herbalists use varying amounts of alcohol to water ratios depending on the compounds they want to extract, but for home use most spirit alcohols, such as brandy, rum or vodka, will work as long as they have at least 40% ABV. Vodka is a good choice as it is clear in colour and has a neutral flavour.

Tinctures can be made with fresh or dried herbs, although fresh is usually the best option, especially when using aromatic herbs, which lose some of their aroma in the drying process. For leaves and flowers, a simple macerated (steeped) tincture will do. For tougher, woodier plant parts, such as dried roots and bark, it is a good idea to make a strong decoction first to break down cell membranes.

For leaves, flowers, fresh roots & berries

Finely chop fresh herbs or crumble dried herbs, place in a wide-mouthed jar and cover with your alcohol of choice, ensuring all plant material is submerged. Label and date the jar and leave for 2–4 weeks in a cool, dark place, shaking the jar every few days.

After 2–4 weeks, strain out and discard the plant material, and pour the liquid tincture into a dark glass bottle. Label and date again.

For tough dried roots, bark & berries

Place the plant material in a saucepan and pour over just enough water to cover. Bring to the boil, then reduce to a gentle simmer for 10–15 minutes. Do not allow the liquid in the pan to dry out completely, but instead reduce to half of the original liquid.

Pour the liquid and plant material into a measuring jug and add 100ml (3½ fl oz) of alcohol for every 100ml (3½ fl oz) of plant and decoction mix (so a 50:50 alcohol to decoction ratio). Pour this into a wide-mouthed jar, label and date and leave to macerate (steep) for 2–4 weeks, shaking every few days.

After 2–4 weeks, strain out and discard the plant material and pour the liquid tincture into a dark glass bottle. Label and date again.

TO USE Take 2–5ml (½–1 teaspoon) of tincture diluted in a little water, juice or tea 1–3 times a day.

SHELF LIFE Up to 2 years in a cool, dark place.

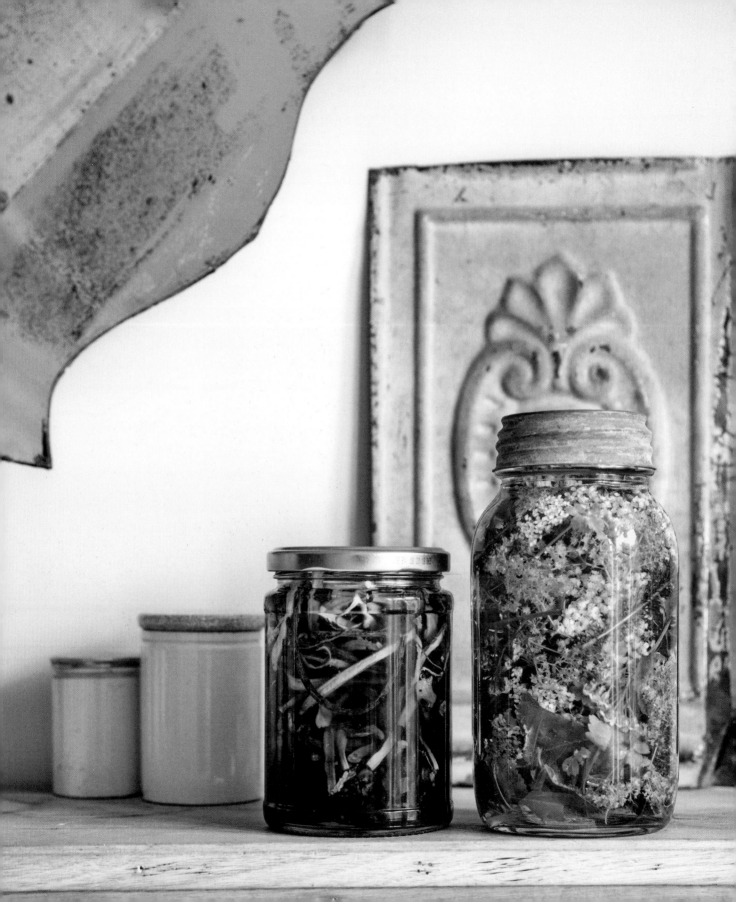

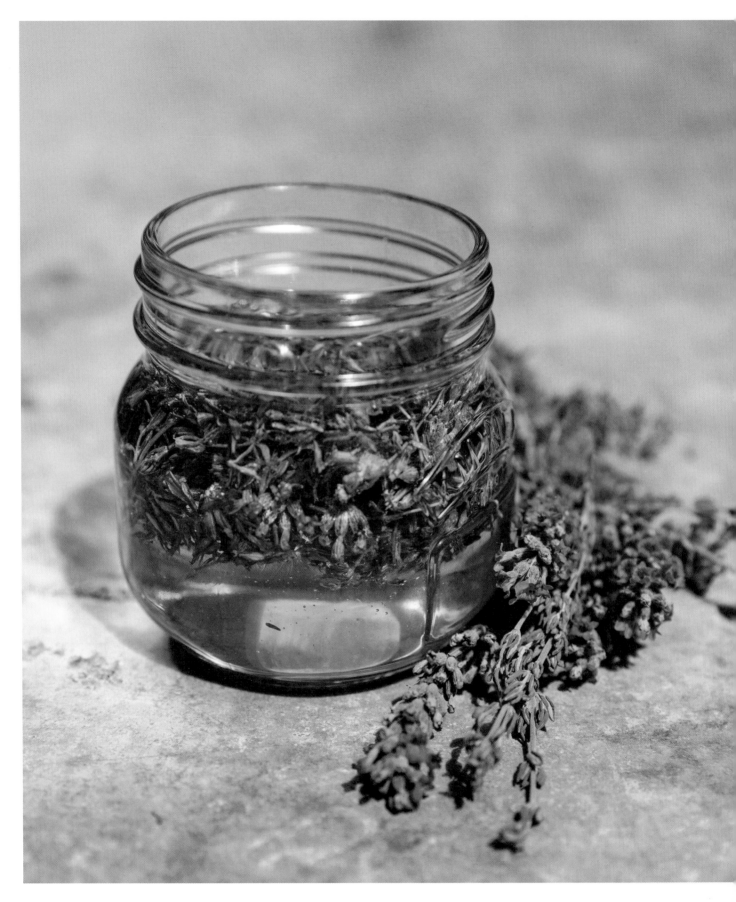

INFUSED HONEY

Honey can extract both water-based and some oil-based plant compounds. Good-quality raw honey contains antimicrobial propolis and healing enzymes and is a medicine in its own right – great for mild infections of the skin and for preparations for sore throats.

Chop your herb of choice finely and place in a sterilised jar. If the honey is set or too thick to pour, gently heat it up by placing its jar in a bowl of warm water. Pour the honey over the herb, ensuring all of the herb is covered. Label and date then leave to infuse for one week, shaking or stirring daily.

After one week, strain out and discard the plant material, reserving the infused honey. Pour or spoon the honey into a wide-mouthed jar. Label and date again.

For a quick method, heat the honey and herbs gently over a low heat for 1 hour and then strain.

TO USE 1 teaspoon can be taken straight off the spoon for sore throats and coughs. Alternatively, mix 1–2 teaspoons into a hot drink.

SHELF LIFE Up to 6 months in a cool, dark place or in the fridge.

GLYCERITES

Glycerites are made in the same way as standard tinctures, but instead of using alcohol they use glycerine, a sweet-tasting, viscous liquid extracted from vegetable sources. They are ideal for children or those who are unable to take alcohol. Glycerites are much thicker than standard tinctures, so are best made using fresh plant material or you will end up with a mass of sticky dried herbs. Because glycerites are high in sugar, they may not be suitable for diabetics.

Finely chop fresh herbs or crumble dried herbs, place in a wide-mouthed jar and cover with glycerine. Label and date the jar and leave for 2–4 weeks in a cool, dark place, shaking the jar every few days.

After 2–4 weeks, strain out and discard the plant material and pour the liquid into a dark glass bottle. Label and date again.

TO USE Take 2–5ml (½–1 teaspoon) in a little water, juice or tea 1–3 times a day.

SHELF LIFE Up to 6 months in a cool, dark place.

SYRUPS

Sugar has long been used to preserve food and medicine for year-round use. There are pros and cons to using sugar for medical preparations. In a world where we massively overconsume sugar-rich foods, the obvious disadvantage is the high calorie content. However, sugar preparations can be beneficial when it comes to those who have lost their appetite due to illness – for instance, with a severe case of tonsillitis, where swallowing solid food is difficult. A herbal syrup will deliver both the medicinal properties of the herb and a few extra calories, giving the body much-needed extra energy to fight off bugs.

Another benefit of syrups is that they are thick – they help to coat irritated membranes, for instance, when the throat is dry from a hacking cough. Sugar also has a slightly demulcent effect, encouraging water to pass through the cell walls in the digestive tract, helping to ease constipation. Honey can be used in place of sugar for this recipe, but it does not preserve as well and is pricey!

SYRUP HERBS

Some herbs need decocting first to make a syrup. These include some tough roots, seeds and fruits, such as elderberry, rosehip and liquorice.

For aromatic and delicate plants, such as elderflower, rose and lemon balm, it's best to make the syrup first and then steep the herbs in the prepared syrup.

Herbal syrup

This recipe can be used for any type of herbal infusion or decoction. Syrups are particularly effective preparations for soothing sore throats and coughs and to relieve constipation.

50g (1¾ oz) fresh or dried herbs
600ml (20 fl oz) water
250–500g (9oz–1lb 2oz) unrefined brown sugar
1–3 teaspoons citric acid (optional for
    preservation and flavour)

Infuse or decoct your herbs as described on pages 12–13. Strain out and discard the plant material. Measure out the strained liquid, and for every 10ml (2 teaspoons) liquid, add 5–10g (⅛–¼oz) sugar. Return to the pan and simmer gently for 10–20 minutes until thickened. The more sugar you add, the longer it will preserve, but watch out: if you boil it for too long with the higher amount of sugar, you may make a sticky jam instead.

Add the citric acid, if using; this balances out the sweetness of the syrup and helps with preservation. Allow to cool and pour into sterilised bottles, label and date.

TO USE 10–30ml (2 teaspoons–1 fl oz) in a cold or warm drink up to 3 times a day, for occasional use.

SHELF LIFE 6–12 months in a cool, dark place. Once open, use within 2 months and store in the fridge.

Herbal pastilles

Herbal pastilles use powdered herbs bound with honey or syrup. Because they are sweet-tasting, they are also a good way of getting herbs into fussy eaters and children.

They are great for sore throats, coughs and digestive problems. Mucilaginous herbs, such as slippery elm or marshmallow root powder, make a great soothing base to which you can add other herbs in a 50:50 ratio. There are two methods to prepare them: either by adding powders to the liquid or vice versa.

herbal powders
honey or glycerine

METHOD ONE
Heat the honey or glycerine gently in a bain-marie (page 24) until runny, then add finely ground herbal powders little by little until a firm paste is formed. Roll into hazelnut-sized balls, place on a baking-parchment-lined tray and and leave to dry fully. You can also speed the process along by drying them in a dehydrator or low oven.

METHOD TWO
Place the herbal powders in a bowl, then add the honey or glycerine little by little until a stiff paste is formed. Roll into hazelnut-sized balls, place on a baking-parchment-lined tray and and leave to dry fully. You can also speed the process along by drying them in a dehydrator or low oven.

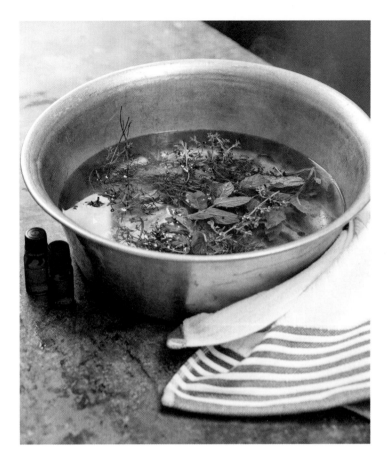

Herbal steam inhalations

Steam inhalations lie somewhere between an internal and an external remedy. They are a great way to deliver aromatic, antimicrobial herbs direct to the sinuses and airways, so are perfect for respiratory conditions such as coughs, colds and sinusitis.

Chop or crush 1 handful of fresh or dried herbs and place in a large heatproof bowl. Boil the kettle and have a large towel at hand. Pour the hot water over the herbs and create a tent over your head with the towel, inhaling the aromatic oils that are lifted into the air through the steam. Alternatively, 5–10 drops of essential oil dropped into the hot water can be used in place of the herbs (see pages 50–51).

EXTERNAL REMEDIES
COMPRESSES & POULTICES   BATHS

Compresses and poultices are easy-to-use herbal remedies, ideal for easing aching joints, sprains, strains and skin conditions.

To make a compress, soak a clean cloth such as a bandage or muslin in a warm or chilled herbal infusion, wring out the excess fluid and place it on the affected area.

Poultices are similar to compresses but involve fresh, soft plant material such as leaves. These can be either crushed and used raw, or crushed and placed in a pan with a little boiling water to cover. The latter will help break open the plant cells, especially if dried herbs are used. Allow to infuse in the water for 5 minutes, then remove from the pan, pour off the excess water and place the herbs between two pieces of muslin or bandage. Place the poultice onto the affected area (as warm as possible, but avoid scalding the skin). Cover with towels to retain the heat and leave on for up to an hour. You can place a hot water bottle on as well to keep the area warm. A traditional poultice uses vinegar and sage (page 101).

Herbal baths, immersions, washes and soaks are a relaxing and healing way to use herbs, although they have fallen out of popular use in recent years. Many indigenous societies use herbal washes in ritual and medicine for their healing properties, such as the use of eucalyptus by the Australian Aboriginal peoples for treating cold and flu symptoms. The famous French herbalist Maurice Mességué treated people with local herbs using hip baths and hand and foot soaks to deliver the medicinal constituents to the body through the skin. Mustard powder foot baths are a European tradition for treating colds and flu; they stimulate circulation to warm and soothe the patient.

Baths & soaks

For relaxing baths and soaks, scented herbs such as lavender, rose, linden and culinary herbs are ideal. However, many other medicinal plants can be used for treating skin, muscles and joints.

1 litre (1¾ pint) water
2–4 handfuls of your herb of choice

Bring the water to the boil in a large pan. Take off the heat, add your plant material and close the lid. Allow to infuse for 15–20 minutes.

TO USE Add the mixture to a bath and soak in it for at least 30 minutes. Alternatively, use part of the liquid in a bowl to soak the hand, wrist or foot for up to 30 minutes, twice a day.

SHELF LIFE The liquid can be kept for up to 4 days in the fridge.

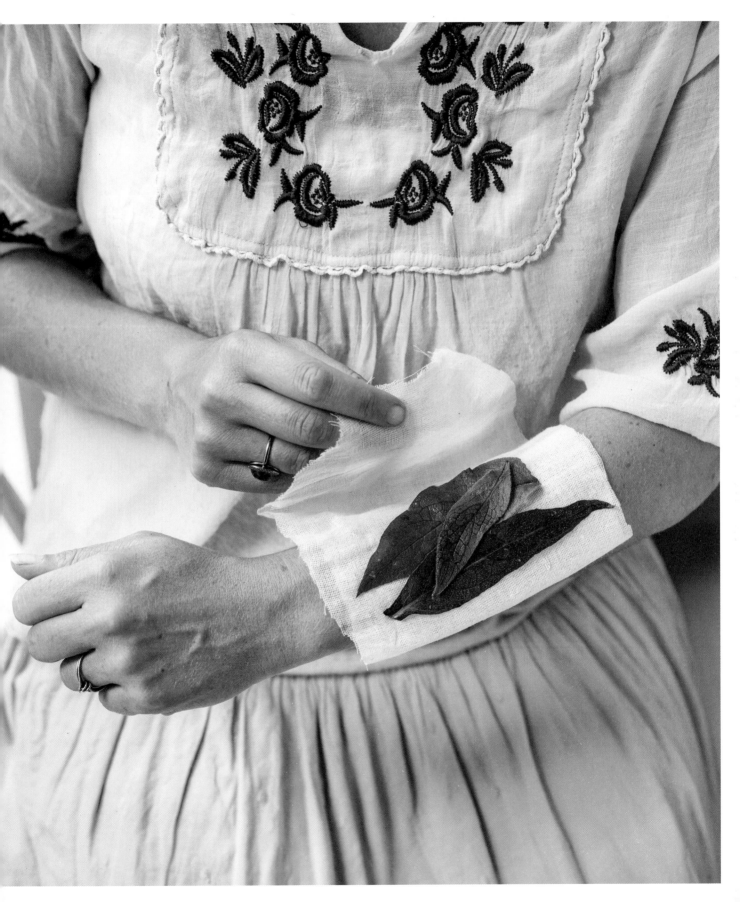

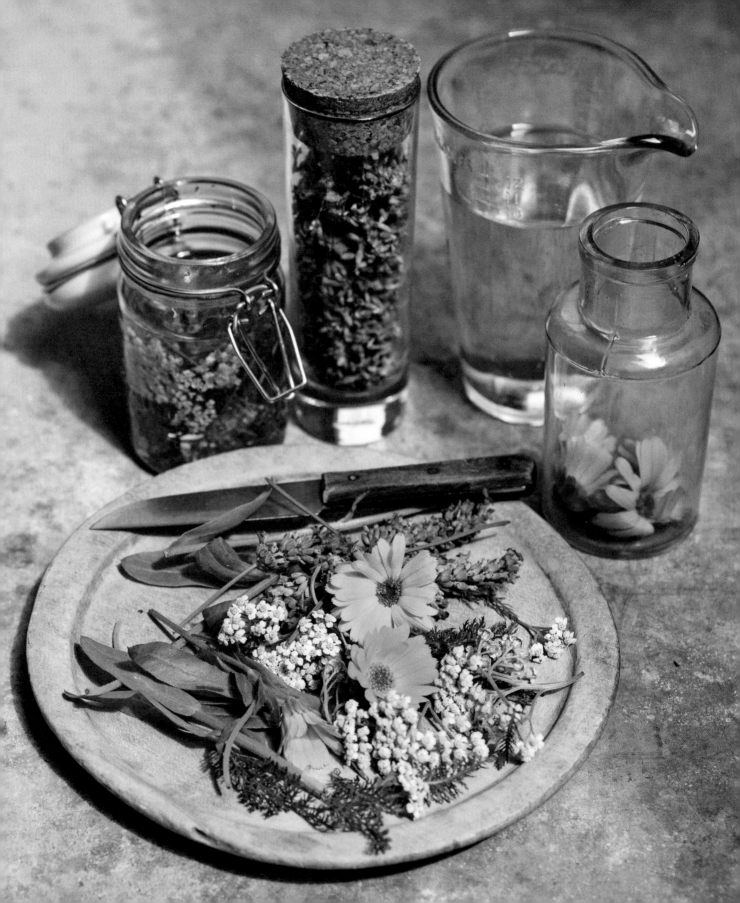

HERBAL INFUSED OILS

Medicinal infused oils are for external use only.

Infusing oils enables the plant's therapeutic benefits to be transferred to an oil that can be stored longer than fresh plant material and in a way that can be conveniently applied to the body. Using an oil also adds moisturising and warming properties that stimulate and soothe when rubbed into the skin. These infused oils are the base to many other external remedies, such as massage oils, bath oils, creams and ointments.

There are a variety of ways to infuse oils with herbs, depending on time constraints. They include infusing slowly using the sun, or using a heat source to extract the plant's properties more quickly.

Infused herbal oil will take on the properties of the plants and usually the colour: calendula infused oil should become a bright orange, St John's wort will become a deep red and comfrey will turn a lovely leaf green. It is at this point that you know your oil is ready to be used.

Traditional sun method

This method takes about 1 month, but needs very little hands-on involvement.

fresh or dried herbs (see box below)
carrier oil

Fill a clean jar loosely with your chosen herb. Pour over enough oil to cover. Try to press down the plant material so it does not float, as this may cause mould growth. You may need to weigh the plant material down with a small clean plate or large, glass marbles. Replace the lid, label and date your mixture. Leave to infuse on a bright windowsill for 1 month. Once infused, strain the oil through a muslin-lined sieve, discarding the herbs, and bottle, label and date.

TIP If you lack a sunny windowsill during the winter period, you can speed up this method by leaving the jar on a radiator for a few days, until the carrier oil has taken on the colour of the herb.

FRESH OR DRIED HERBS?

FRESH HERBS can be used to create infused oils. However, because they contain water, when added to oil they can cause it to become rancid or mouldy and so need careful processing. The quick-heated methods (page 24) are best when using fresh plant material. It is always best to remove excess water by first wilting your plant for a day or so. After infusing your herbal oil, and once the herb material has been strained off, any remaining water should drop to the bottom of the oil and can be siphoned off. When straining the herb from the oil, DO NOT squeeze the herb, as this will extract more water and increase the likelihood of the oil spoiling. If the oil remains cloudy, gently heat the oil again to evaporate any water that remains.

DRIED HERBS are easier to use and less likely to spoil when making infused oils, but to obtain the best-quality oil, use herbs that have been freshly dried. This maintains the best properties of the plant yet removes the issue of water contamination.

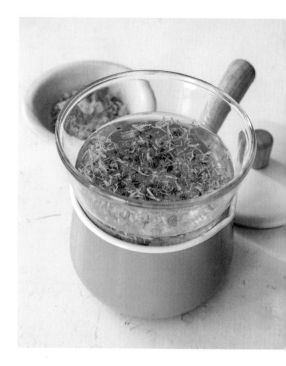

THE DIFFERENCE BETWEEN ESSENTIAL OILS, CARRIER OILS, BUTTERS AND INFUSED OILS

ESSENTIAL OILS, including lavender, rose, orange and frankincense, are extracted from the aromatic oils that naturally occur in plants, usually in leaves, flowers and from some resins. Think of the scent of a lavender flower; lavender essential oil is that scent extracted (through steam distillation) and captured in a bottle. Essential oils are potent oils that are concentrated plant chemicals and you will only ever need to use a few drops at a time and usually diluted. For more on essential oils, see pages 50–51.

CARRIER OILS, also known as base oils, include olive, sunflower, almond or jojoba oils. These are oils extracted from the part of the plant that contains fats (heavy, non-aromatic oils) and are pressed out of the plant. These are mild and can be used alone as simple moisturisers, or as a base in which to dilute essential oils or infuse herbs.

BUTTERS, such as shea, cocoa or mango seed butters, are similar to carrier oils but are solid at room temperature. They can be melted easily and also act as moisturisers, or as a base in which to mix essential oils or infuse herbs.

INFUSED OILS are carrier oils or butters infused with the medicinal, oil-soluble properties of herbs. Examples include calendula, St John's wort and comfrey oils.

Quick pan/bain-marie method

This method will result in herbal oil after just a few hours' preparation. This is easily made in a bain-marie if you have one, or use a pan and heatproof bowl to make your own homemade bain-marie/double boiler.

fresh or dried herbs (see box, page 23)
carrier oil
water

Put the herbs in a heatproof bowl and cover with oil. Set the bowl over a pan of gently simmering water; it should sit on top of the pan without touching the water. Allow the herbs to infuse into the oil for about 2–3 hours. Keep checking the level of the water in the pan and top up as needed, taking care of any escaping steam.

If you would like a stronger infused oil, strain out the oil, and if using dried herbs, squeeze out as much oil out as you can. Discard the old plant material and refresh your oil with a new batch of herbs. Repeat the first step.

Once the oil is infused, strain out and discard the plant material again. You may require a muslin-lined sieve to remove all the small particles. Pour the infused oil into jars or bottles, label and date.

Slow-cooker method

A slow cooker with a 'keep warm' setting is required; this keeps a low constant heat without the need for topping up water, as needed in the quick pan method.

carrier oil
fresh or dried herbs (see box, page 23)

Place the carrier oil and herbs in your slow-cooker bowl. The oil should cover the herbs, but not be excessive. Place the lid on if the herbs are dry, but leave the lid off if they are fresh, to allow the water to evaporate. Leave on the 'keep warm' setting for a few hours or overnight.

If you would like a stronger infused oil, strain out the oil, and if using dried herbs, squeeze as much oil out as you can. Discard the old plant material and refresh your oil with a new batch of herbs. Repeat the first step.

Once the oil is infused, strain out and discard the plant material again. You may require a muslin-lined sieve to remove all the small particles. Pour the infused oil into jars or bottles, label and date.

SHELF LIFE FOR ALL METHODS OF INFUSED OIL
Up to 1 year in a clean, airtight container stored in a cool dark place. To preserve the oils, add 1% vitamin E oil to your total amount of finished infused oil.

Creams are similar to ointments, but have the addition of a water-based element. Oil and water don't mix, so emulsifiers such as beeswax or emulsifying wax are also needed. This brings the healing herbal constituents that are extracted in both water and oil to the creams, but creams are more cooling than ointments. Ideal for cuts, itchy rashes and to create soothing body creams.

50ml (2 fl oz) herbal infused oil (page 23)
10g (¼ oz) cocoa butter
10g (¼ oz) beeswax
5g (⅛ oz) emulsifying wax
20ml (4 teaspoons) herbal tincture (page 14)
30ml (1fl oz) herbal infusion (pages 12–13)
20 drops essential oil (this can be a mixture of your choice)

In a large pan, place two wide-mouthed jars in 5cm (2in) of gently heating (not quite simmering) water. In one jar, place the herbal infused oil, cocoa butter, beeswax and allow to melt. In the other jar, melt the emulsifying wax with the tincture and infusion. Take care not to allow the pan to boil.

Take both jars off the heat and allow to cool slightly. Both jars need to be at the same temperature for mixing, so if the infusion mix cools a little quicker, return to the heat. Gradually and very slowly, drop by drop, pour the infusion/tincture mix into the oil mixture, whisking quickly (an electric mixer works best) until thoroughly combined and cooled. This will create a creamy consistency. At this point you can whisk in the essential oils. Spoon into sterilised jars, label and date.

SHELF LIFE Store in the fridge for up to 6 months.

TIP For a vegan cream, replace the beeswax with half the amount of caranauba or candelilla wax.

OINTMENTS & BALMS

The words 'ointment' and 'balm' are often used inter-changeably, but are generally oil-based remedies created using herbal infused oils set with butters or waxes. They are warming and best used for dry skin, or for bringing warmth to areas such as aching joints and muscles. They are best avoided on itchy, hot rashes such as eczema or hives where a cream with added cooling water properties would be better indicated (page 123).

herbal infused oil (page 23)
beeswax (see box for ratios)
essential oils (20–60 drops per 100ml/3½ fl oz)
    see pages 50–1 for guidance

Place your herbal infused oil and beeswax in a heatproof bowl over a pan of gently simmering water. Mix gently until the beeswax has dissolved.

Remove the bowl from the heat and allow to cool for a few minutes before mixing in any essential oils with a metal spoon or knitting needle. Allowing the oil to cool slightly reduces the chance of the essential oils evaporating away.

Pour the liquid into a warm jug, then pour into jars. Allow to set, then place on the lids, clean the outside of the jars to remove any trace of oil, label and date.

SHELF LIFE Up to 1 year stored in a cool, dark place.

TIP For a vegan alternative, replace the beeswax with half the amount of candelilla or caranauba wax.

Herbal infused butters such as shea or cocoa, which are solid at room temperature, can also be infused for a ready-made balm instead of using a runny carrier oil. Once strained and cooled, the butter will naturally set, making a firm ointment.

LINIMENTS

Also known as an embrocation, a liniment is a rubbing liquid for easing aches and pains, usually made with an oil or alcohol base, such as an infused herbal oil or tincture. They can be mixed at a 50:50 oil to alcohol ratio. Shake thoroughly before use. See page 14 for an example.

OIL TO WAX RATIOS FOR OINTMENTS & BALMS

25g (1oz) beeswax to 100ml (3½ fl oz) oil – firm ointment
20g (¾ oz) beeswax to 100ml (3½ fl oz) oil – medium ointment
15g (½ oz) beeswax to 100ml (3½ fl oz) oil – soft ointment

If you live in a warmer country, you may need to add a little extra beeswax to keep the ointment set, or store in the fridge.

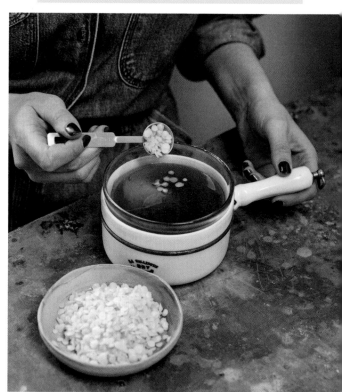

FLORAL WATERS

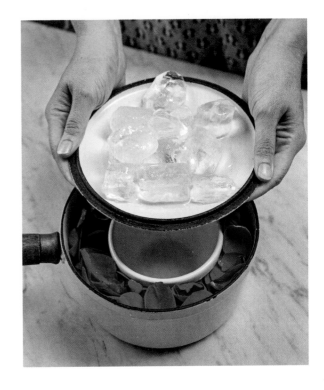

Floral waters, also known as hydrosols or hydrolats, are produced during the essential-oil-making process, where steam is used to draw out the volatile oils from aromatic herbs. This steam is then condensed and the resulting liquid is the aromatic floral water, infused with both water- and oil-based plant compounds. In mass production, using very large stills called alembics, the essential oil floats on the top of this water and is siphoned off. A smaller home set-up will not produce essential oils, but does produce lovely, medicinal floral waters. Dried or fresh herbs can be used.

Although floral waters can be taken internally in small quantities, they are used here in external remedies, as they are excellent for skin-healing preparations and to make room and body sprays for calming anxiety and aiding sleep.

The following method enables distilling using everyday kitchen equipment. You'll need a saucepan with a dome-shaped lid that you can turn upside-down; the handle of the lid should be non-absorbent. You will also need a heatproof bowl small enough to slip inside the pan, leaving a 3–5cm (1¼in–2in) gap around the edges. This is best suited for aromatic flowers and leaves such as lavender, rose, lemon balm and rosemary, to name a few.

500ml (18 fl oz) filtered water (plus extra for topping up)
a few handfuls of fresh or dried aromatic herbs
plenty of ice cubes

Pour the filtered water into the saucepan. Place the heatproof bowl in the centre of the pan, then place your flowers around the outside of the bowl, so that they cover the water. Put the lid, upside-down, onto the saucepan. The lid handle should be pointing into the empty bowl.

Bring the pan to a gentle simmer. Fill the inverted lid with ice cubes, then allow the steam to condense for approximately 30 minutes, ensuring the pan does not boil dry. The evaporating water, along with the aromatic properties of the plant material, will hit the upside-down pan lid and condense back into the bowl because the lid is iced. As the ice melts, top it up with more ice, pouring away the melted ice before you add more. This will not make copious amounts of floral water, but enough for personal use.

TIP There is a 'quick' version of floral water on page 131, which uses essential oils and alcohol to disperse the scent evenly through the water to create scented room and body sprays.

CULINARY HERBS

Culinary herbs and spices make great medicines. When illness strikes, it is really useful to know about remedies you can rustle up using ingredients commonly found in the kitchen cupboard or a local supermarket.

ANISEED/ANISE – *Pimpinella anisum*
Similar to dill and fennel in its herbal actions, aniseed is a great digestive, helping to relieve spasms in the gut and lessen flatulence and bloating when used in infusions or chewed. A syrup of aniseed is an age-old remedy for cutting through mucus in the chest and relieving coughs. Like fennel, it can ease colic in babies when given as a tea to the nursing mother and can promote breast milk production (see recipe on page 165). Chewing the seeds can help with bad breath.
CONDITIONS *Coughs, colds, colic, weak digestion, flatulence, poor appetite, scant breast milk production*
RECIPES *Fennel & mint after-dinner pyramids (page 69); Herbal cough drops (page 115); Mothers' tea (page 165)*

BAY – *Laurus nobilis*
Bay is warming and stimulating to the digestive system and can be added to food to aid digestion. The warming qualities of bay are handy for aching muscles, joints and bad backs. To warm up and heal achey muscles, try an infused oil or balm of bay leaf.
CONDITIONS *Bad back, muscle and joint aches and pains*
RECIPES *Bone broth (page 76); Vegan mushroom broth (page 78); Ache-ease liniment (page 97)*

BLACK PEPPER – *Piper nigrum*
Black pepper is warming to the digestive system. It aids the absorption of other herbs and foods, particularly turmeric, where piperine (a constituent in pepper) helps the absorption of curcuminoids (a group of beneficial antioxidant phytochemicals in turmeric). The essential oil is ideal for adding to warming rubs and massage balms, though a little goes a long way so use sparingly.
CONDITIONS *Aching muscles and joints, poor digestion, poor circulation*
RECIPES *Elderberry Liqueur (page 82); Fire cider (page 82); Ache-ease liniment (page 96); Elderberry syrup (page 111)*

CARDAMOM – *Elletaria cardamomum*
Making an infusion with, or chewing, cardamom seeds helps sweeten the breath, aids digestion, flatulence and coughs. A tincture of the crushed pods and seeds makes a numbing blend that can be used as a gargle, spray or mouthwash for sore throats, mouth ulcers and toothache (page 14). Cardamom is an uplifting herb, the smell alone can help lessen frayed nerves, so add the seeds to infusions, chai or add the essential oil to massage balms. In Ayurveda, it is used for improving stress and headaches associated with stress.
CONDITIONS *Bad breath, flatulence, coughs, sore throats, mouth ulcers, toothache, anxiety, low mood, weak digestion, convalescence*
RECIPES *Elderberry liqueur (page 82); Relaxing massage bars (page 93); Cardamom, rose & linden cocoa (page 95); Elderberry syrup (page 111); Sore throat gargle (page 119)*

CHILLI/CAYENNE – *Capsicum annuum*
Chilli can stimulate appetite and also make us feel more satiated after a meal at the same time. The deeply warming action of chilli boosts a sluggish digestive system, helping the body to digest, break down and in turn absorb the nutrients from food more efficiently. It is a circulatory stimulant, opening up even the tiny blood vessels, allowing heat to permeate through the body so it is great for poor circulation.

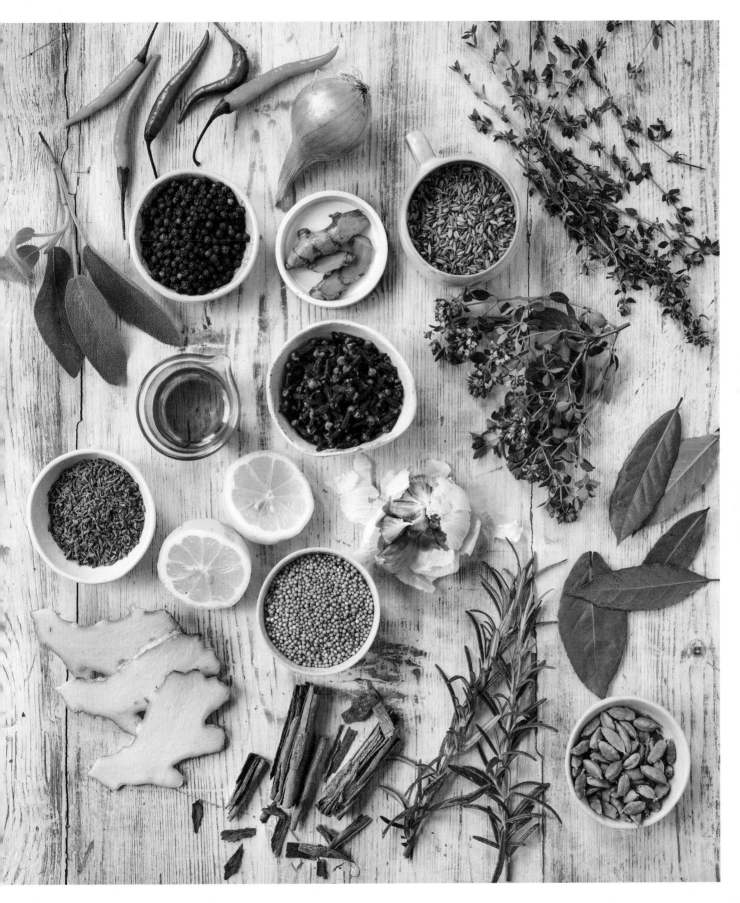

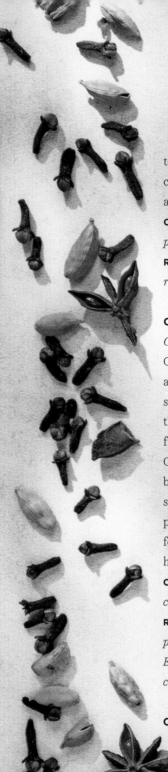

The warming properties of chilli can be used to help reduce pain. Warming rubs (see page 96) can be used to help soothe aching muscles, joints and abdominal discomfort, such as period pain.

CONDITIONS *Poor circulation, muscle and joint pain, back ache, poor digestion*

RECIPES *Fire cider (page 82); Chilli & ginger joint rub (page 96)*

CINNAMON – *Cinnamomum zeylanicum, C. verum*

Cinnamon is warming, drying and antimicrobial and is used for clearing mucus in the lungs and sinuses in coughs, colds and flu. It is stimulating to the circulatory system, benefiting those who suffer from poor circulation, such as cold hands and feet. Cinnamon powder lends sweetness to foods and beverages without the need for sugar. Research suggests that taking ½–1 teaspoon of cinnamon powder daily (as capsules, infusions or mixed into food) could help to balance blood sugar levels and help to lower high cholesterol.

CONDITIONS *Weak digestion, infections, high cholesterol, colds, coughs, flu*

RECIPES *Herbal hot toddy (page 74); Elderberry pastilles (page 81); Elderberry liqueur (page 82); Elderberry syrup (page 111); Ashwagandha, flax & chia seed pudding (page 152)*

CLOVES – *Syzygium aromaticum*

Cloves contain eugenol, an anaesthetic, antiviral and antiseptic volatile oil. For quick relief of toothache, simply chew on a clove bud; the antimicrobial effects may also help with any underlying tooth infection.

Alternatively, soak a small piece of cotton with 1 drop of clove essential oil. For children, dilute in ½ teaspoon of carrier oil and place carefully over a painful tooth or mouth ulcer (see pages 46–47). For sore throats or mouth ulcers, a tincture of cloves can be diluted 1:5 with water and used as a mouthwash or mouth spray.

RECIPES *Herbal hot toddy (page 74); Elderberry liqueur (page 82); Four thieves vinegar (page 85); Elderberry syrup (page 111); Sore throat gargle (page 119)*

FENNEL – *Foeniculum vulgare*

Fennel is a top digestive herb. An infusion of the seeds gives an effective remedy for flatulence and bloating. Fennel contains both sweet (soothing) and bitter (stimulating) compounds – try chewing the seeds after a heavy meal for improving digestion. The sweet taste and gentle action makes it a great remedy for children's tummy ache or trapped wind. For kids, try it in a weak infusion flavoured with lemon and/or honey. Fennel tea can also be used to encourage breast milk production and is taken by nursing mothers to improve milk flow and to ease colic in babies (see page 165).

CONDITIONS *Bad breath, colic, flatulence, nausea, scanty breast milk production, tummy ache*

RECIPES *After-dinner tea (page 65); Fennel & mint after-dinner pyramids (page 69); Mother's tea (page 165)*

GARLIC – *Allium sativum*

Garlic has a wide range of antimicrobial compounds, including allicin and sulphur compounds. Much of garlic's antimicrobial compounds are excreted through the lungs, meaning they get exactly where they need to be for chest infections, such as bronchitis, colds and flu. It can be eaten regularly as a preventative during cold and flu season. The sulphur compounds in garlic are responsible both for its strong odour and many of its medicinal effects. These compounds are broken down with cooking but are increased when garlic cloves are crushed, so it is best to crush garlic 5 minutes before use and consume it raw when using it as a medicine. Try it raw in bruschetta, stirred into soups or whizzed into salad dressings. If garlic breath is something you want to avoid, try chewing on some fresh parsley or fennel seeds after eating it. Inulin, a type of dietary fibre found in garlic, acts as a prebiotic (food source for good bacteria in the gut). This, combined with its antimicrobial actions, makes garlic great for those with tummy troubles and food poisoning. Studies have shown that regular consumption of raw garlic may help to protect the cardiovascular system and lower both high cholesterol and high blood pressure.

CONDITIONS *Cough, colds, flu, food poisoning, poor gut health, fungal infections, bacterial infections, viril infections*

RECIPES *Nettle soup (page 54); Bone broth (page 76); Mushroom tonic soup (page 77); Fire cider (page 82); Four theives vinegar (page 85); Nettle & mushroom concentrate powder (page 103); Three herb & onion cough syrup (page 112); Garlic & mullein ear oil (page 140)*

GINGER – *Zingiber officinale*

Ginger is an excellent remedy for all kinds of nausea, including morning sickness in early pregnancy and travel sickness. It is a deeply heating and permeating herb, it lends its warming qualities to the digestive and circulatory systems, in turn aiding the absorption of many herbs and nutrients it is used with. It is a great herb to add to teas, tinctures and remedies for people who have slow digestion, poor circulation or where their illness is made worse in cold conditions. Ginger helps to clear mucus in the chest and throat, making it a great remedy for coughs, colds and sore throats.

CONDITIONS *Nausea, poor circulation, poor digestion, coughs, sore throats, cold and flu*

RECIPES *Bitter digestive spray (page 66); Hangover powders (page 73); Herbal hot toddy (page 74); Elderberry liqueur (page 82); Fire cider (page 82); Chilli & ginger joint rub (page 96); Muscle ease tincture (page 99); Cold & flu infusion (page 108); Elderberry syrup (page 111); Herbal cough drops (page 115); Ginger & honey throat melts (page 120); Cramp drops (page 150); Crystallised ginger & lemon (page 159); Happy mummy spray (page 164)*

LEMONS – *Citrus limon*

Lemons are high in vitamin C, which is beneficial to the immune system. The tart acidity of lemon juice is great for cutting through mucus – combine it with honey or herbal syrups for sore throats, coughs and colds. Lemon peel contains antimicrobial volatile oils which can be employed in household cleaning products and beauty products to clean and clear problematic oily or spotty skin.

CONDITIONS *Sore throats, coughs, colds, acne, oily skin*

RECIPES *Herbal hot toddy (page 74); Fire cider (page 82); Spot banishing gel (page 122); Nourishing skin cream (acne) (page 123); Herbal hair rinse (blonde) (page 134); Castor oil hair-conditioning mask (page 137); Aftershave gel (page 144); Crystallised ginger & lemon (page 159)*

MUSTARD – *Brassica alba, B. hirta, B. nigra, B. junica*

Mustard foot baths are an old remedy for coughs, colds, chills, and headaches, tired feet and aching joints and muscles. To make a mustard foot bath, mix 2 tablespoons mustard powder with 2 litres (3½ pints) hot water, allow to cool to a comfortable temperature and soak the feet for at least 20 minutes. Mustard poultices and plasters for the chest made using a thick paste of mustard powder mixed with hot water are also an age-old remedy for coughs and colds – be careful though, they are very warming on the skin so best avoided in young children and those with sensitive skin! It is best to cover the area of the skin that will be treated with oil first and create a layer of muslin or bandage between the mustard and the skin. Remove after 5–10 minutes.

CONDITIONS *Poor circulation, colds, flu, coughs, headache, muscle and joint pain*

RECIPES *Warming hand and foot bath (page 57); Herbal muscle soak (page 100)*

OLIVE – *Olea europaea*

Cold-pressed olive oil makes a great carrier for infusing with other herbs and essential oils. It is antibacterial and healing to the skin when used externally. Try infusing olive oil with dried rosemary for a scalp-stimulating hair treatment to soothe dandruff and lacklustre hair (page 137). Olive leaf is antimicrobial – you can buy it in extract form or use the leaves to make a strong tea or decoction to wash wounds and skin infections, including fungal infections such as athlete's foot. Olive leaf tea or extract has protective effects on the cardiovascular system and can help lower slightly raised blood pressure. A teaspoon of olive oil can be used for soothing dry, irritated sore throats and coughs.

CONDITIONS *Eczema, dandruff, dull hair, skin infections, fungal infections, athlete's foot, high blood pressure, coughs and sore throats*

RECIPES *Lemon balm & St John's wort infused oil (page 87); Comfrey balm (page 104); Garlic & mullein ear oil (page 140); Nappy rash ointment (page 169)*

ONION – *Allium cepa*

Onions have an antimicrobial effect on the lungs, helping to kill bacteria and cut through mucus in coughs and respiratory infections. A super-quick and effective cough syrup can be made with onions and sugar (see page 112). Onion juice can be used for mild skin infections, warts, insect bites and burns or an onion poultice for splinters. Like garlic, onions contain dietary fibre that feed good bacteria in the gut, making it a great food to eat to maintain general gut health.

CONDITIONS *Coughs, sore throats, insect bites, cuts, warts, poor gut health*

RECIPES *Nettle soup (page 54); Bone broth (page 76); Mushroom tonic soup (page 77); Vegan mushroom broth (page 78); Fire cider (page 82); Three herb & onion cough syrup (page 112)*

OREGANO AND MARJORAM – *Origanum vulgare,*
O. majorana

Oregano and marjoram are closely related and used interchangeably in herbal medicine. They are powerfully antimicrobial, particularly for fungal conditions. A tea made from the bruised fresh or dry leaves can be used as a wash for skin infections, wounds and thrush.

CONDITIONS *Sore throat, infection, bronchitis, dull headaches, cough, indigestion, fungal conditions, athlete's foot, ringworm, thrush*

RECIPES *Antimicrobial gel (page 37); Wound wash (page 38); Three herb & onion cough syrup (page 112)*

CONDITIONS *Hot flushes, poor memory, sore throats, aching muscles and joints, poor hair growth*

RECIPES *Wound wash (page 38); Four thieves vinegar (page 85); Three herb & onion cough syrup (page 112); Herbal hair rinse (page 135)*

THYME – *Thymus vulgaris*

Thyme is a highly aromatic and antimicrobial herb. The tincture, infusion or diluted essential oil can be applied to minor cuts and bacterial and fungal skin infections. Thyme has long been valued as an anti-infective for the respiratory and digestive systems, so is particularly suited to coughs and upset digestions.

CONDITIONS *Coughs, colds, flu, fungal infections, athlete's foot, ringworm*

RECIPES *Antimicrobial gel (page 37); Wound wash (page 38); Nettle iron drops (page 56); Oral rehydration salts (page 71); Elderberry pastilles (page 81); Fire cider (page 82); Four thieves vinegar (page 85); Decongestant chest rub (page 107); Three herb & onion cough syrup (page 112); Herbal cough drops (page 115); Nasal wash (page 121); Spot banishing gel (page 122); Antifungal powder (page 146)*

TURMERIC – *Curcuma longa*

Turmeric is one of the most anti-inflammatory and antioxidant herbs in the kitchen cupboard. In Ayurvedic medicine, turmeric has been used as a longevity herb. It is often taken for inflammatory conditions such as rheumatoid arthritis. It can be used in fresh or dried (powdered) form. One of the main medicinal and anti-inflammatory compounds in turmeric, curcumin, is particularly well absorbed when combined with fats and black pepper. Take turmeric powder in a little coconut oil, nut milks, curries or in capsules with a pinch of black pepper added. A paste made from turmeric and water or honey can be applied to inflammatory skin conditions such as acne spots and psoriasis.

CONDITIONS *Rheumatoid arthritis, acne, ageing, circulatory support*

RECIPES *Hangover powders (page 73); Fire cider (page 82) Antifungal powder (page 146); Ashwagandha, flax & chia seed pudding (page 152);*

FIRST AID

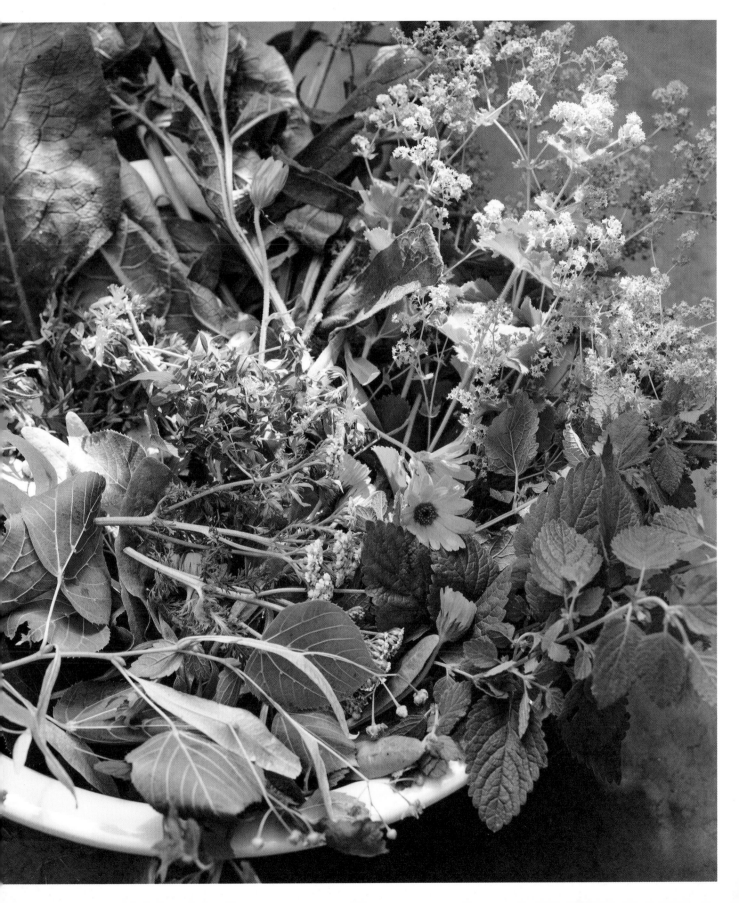

HERBAL FIRST-AID KIT

Basic guidance is provided here, but for medical emergencies see a doctor. For minor first-aid situations, consult an up-to-date first-aid manual or healthcare practitioner for best practice.

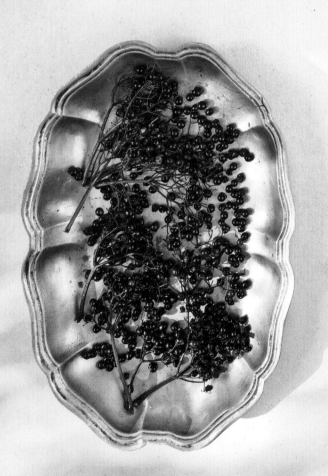

Ten all-round first-aid recipes that can be made in advance for easy access when you need them.

REMEDY	USE
Healing ointment *(page 38)*	*Rashes, cuts, insect bites and stings, eczema*
Comfrey infused oil or balm *(page 104)*	*Broken bones, sprains, strains, bruising, muscle/joint aches and pains*
Anti-allergy infusion *(page 116)*	*Hayfever, sinusitis, eczema, general allergies, fevers, colds and flu*
Itchy-eye cooler cubes *(page 118)*	*Itchy, hayfever-swollen eyes, sunburn, insect bites and stings, rashes*
Skin-soothing gel *(page 44)*	*Minor burns, sunburn, rashes, insect bites and stings*
Elderberry syrup or liqueur *(pages 82 and 111)*	*Coughs, sore throats, colds, flu, general infections*
Sore throat gargle *(page 119)*	*Sore throats, mouth ulcers*
Chamomile and linden infusion or tincture *(page 142)*	*Anxiety, insomnia, colds, flu, indigestion*
Fig and prune syrup *(page 63)*	*Constipation*
Bramble-stop tea *(page 72)*	*Diarrhoea, sore throats*

GRAZES, CUTS AND WOUNDS

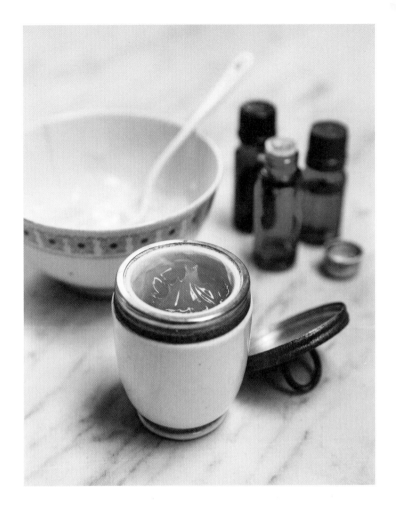

Always rinse out cuts and wounds as soon as they happen to dislodge dirt or bacteria. For simple cuts, encourage skin healing with the use of vulnerary (wound-healing) and anti-infective herbs to help prevent infection. Yarrow leaf poultice has been used to stop bleeding wounds. Try healing creams and balms using the herbs below.

EXTERNAL HERBS *Calendula, lavender, self-heal, St John's wort, yarrow, comfrey (avoid using comfrey for deep cuts as it can quickly heal the top layer of the wound and trap in infection)*

RECIPES *Wound wash and Healing ointment (page 38); Chickweed, plantain and aloe poultice (page 40)*

Antimicrobial gel

Great for preventing infection in cuts, grazes, bites and other skin irritations, this herbal antiseptic gel is a must for any herbal first-aid cupboard and can be tailored to either antifungal or antibacterial versions.

ANTIBACTERIAL VERSION
80g (3oz) aloe vera gel
20ml (4 teaspoons) thyme tincture
10 drops lavender essential oil
10 drops yarrow essential oil

ANTIFUNGAL VERSION
80g (3oz) aloe vera gel
10ml (2 teaspoons) thyme tincture
10ml (2 teaspoons) myrrh tincture
10 drops oregano or thyme essential oil
10 drops eucalyptus or tea tree essential oil

Mix together all the ingredients for your chosen version in a jar and shake well. Label and date the jar.

TO USE Apply to affected area as required.

SHELF LIFE Up to 6 months in a cool, dark place.

Wound wash

This strong infusion of vulnerary (wound-healing) and anti-infective herbs (use fresh or dried) makes an ideal wash or compress for cuts, bumps and grazes.

1 tablespoon fresh or dried vulnerary herbs (see below)
1 tablespoon fresh or dried antimicrobial herbs (see below)
200ml (⅓ pint) boiling water
½ teaspoon salt

VULNERARY HERBS	ANTIMICROBIAL HERBS
Plantain	Lavender
Calendula	Thyme
Self-heal	Rosemary
Comfrey	Sage
Chickweed	Eucalyptus
St John's wort	Oregano
Gotu kola	

Steep your chosen herbs in the boiling water for 10–15 minutes.

Strain out and discard the herbs, then add the salt to the liquid. Allow to cool to body temperature.

Alternatively, dilute the same herbal tinctures in water and use as a wash: 10% tincture to 90% water.

TO USE Use to wash wounds or as a compress (page 20).

SHELF LIFE Use immediately.

Healing ointment

This simple ointment is a remedy for skin irritations, cuts and grazes. Calendula and plantain encourage skin healing and scab formation, while powerfully anti-inflammatory yarrow essential oil reduces the risk of infection through its antimicrobial action.

2 teaspoons beeswax
50ml (2 fl oz) calendula infused oil
20ml (4 teaspoons) plantain infused oil
10ml (2 teaspoons) St John's wort tincture
15 drops yarrow or lavender
   essential oil

Heat the beeswax, calendula and plantain infused oils in a bain-marie (see page 24) until the beeswax has melted. Add the St John's wort tincture drop by drop, whisking continuously until combined well.

Remove from the heat and allow to cool a little. Add your preferred essential oil and stir through. Pour into dark glass jars, label and date.

TO USE Apply to affected areas as needed.

SHELF LIFE Up to 6 months in an airtight container.

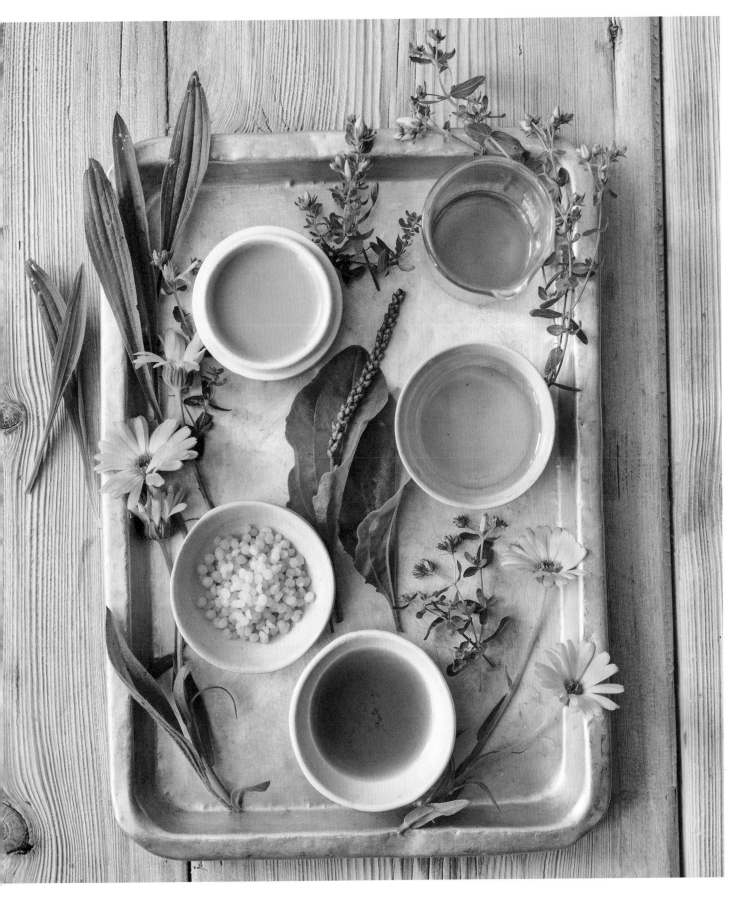

ITCHY RASH

Itchy rashes are usually caused by an allergy, insect bite or irritating plant, such as stinging nettles. When mild they can be treated with simple skin-soothing herbs. Herbal first-aid treatment aims to bring down inflammation and itching by applying anti-inflammatory and anti-allergy herbs in the form of creams, washes, poultices, infused oils and balms.

INTERNAL HERBS *Nettle, plantain, elderflower*

EXTERNAL HERBS *Chickweed, oats, calendula, plantain, lavender, chamomile, aloe vera*

RECIPES *Chickweed, plantain & aloe poultice (see right); Skin-soothing gel (page 44); Oaty bath balls (page 129)*

Chickweed, plantain & aloe poultice

Chickweed and plantain are the go-to plants for soothing itchy rashes. When combined with aloe, this cooling remedy will calm inflammation and reduce the need to scratch.

1 medium-sized aloe leaf (20–30cm/8–12in long)
   or 30ml (1 fl oz) shop-bought aloe gel
5 large plantain leaves
a small handful of fresh chickweed

If using fresh aloe, cut the leaf in half and scoop out the clear, inner gel. Place all the ingredients in a blender or pestle and mortar and whizz or grind until you have a smooth paste.

TO USE Apply the mixture to the affected area, cover with a clean muslin or bandage and wrap with clingfilm. If hot or cold alleviates the itch, apply a hot or cold compress accordingly.

SHELF LIFE Use immediately.

ALLERGIES

INSECT BITES & STINGS

For simple allergy symptoms, such as sneezing and itchy eyes, as experienced in seasonal hayfever, or dust allergies, drink infusions or tinctures of traditional herbs used for their anti-inflammatory, anti-allergy properties.

INTERNAL HERBS *Nettle, plantain, elderflower, chamomile, eyebright*

EXTERNAL HERBS *(compresses for itchy hives/swollen eyes) Eyebright, chickweed, aloe vera, witch hazel*

RECIPES *Anti-allergy infusion (page 116); Itchy-eye cooler cubes (page 118)*

CAUTION For sudden and severe allergies, such as anaphylaxis, which can be life-threatening, medical treatment must be sought immediately. Symptoms can include, but are not limited to, any or all of the following:

- swelling of the body, but particularly the face and mouth, which can restrict breathing
- inflamed or overly pale skin
- rashes such as hives, itchiness, particularly full-body
- dizziness and fainting
- stomach pain, diarrhoea or vomiting
- weak, rapid pulse

BROKEN BONES & FRACTURES
See page 104.

Make compresses or poultices with a strong infusion of the fresh or dried herbs below, as well as drinking a few cups of the Anti-allergy hayfever infusion recipe on page 116. Seek medical help if the patient has a severe reaction, problems breathing or has previous records of anaphylaxis.

EXTERNAL HERBS *Plantain, chickweed, cleavers, marshmallow leaf or root, calendula, slippery elm*

RECIPES *Antimicrobial gel (page 37); Healing ointment (page 38); Chickweed, plantain & aloe poultice (see opposite); Peppermint roll-on (page 42); Skin-soothing gel (page 44); Anti-allergy infusion (page 116)*

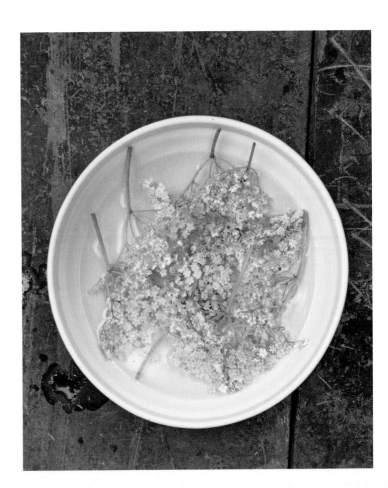

HEADACHES

Headaches occur for myriad reasons; they could be due to eyestrain, dehydration, hormonal imbalance, digestive issues, to name just a few. So treat the headache accordingly: if you find you suffer from headaches when you are stressed, have some relaxing herbal teas to hand; if your headaches are associated with neck tension, use tension-relaxing herbs such as linden, chamomile and hawthorn. For those that suffer from ongoing headaches or migraines, it is important to get to the root cause of the issue by seeing a herbalist. A general herbal remedy to alleviate simple headaches uses peppermint essential oil (see the Peppermint roll-on recipe, right).

INTERNAL HERBS *Linden flower, cramp bark, meadowsweet, wood betony, lemon balm, valerian, vervain, feverfew*

ESSENTIAL OILS *Peppermint, lavender*

RECIPES *Peppermint roll-on (see right); Sage vinegar compress (page 101)*

Peppermint roll-on

This aromatherapy roll-on uses pain-relieving lavender and cooling peppermint and eucalyptus essential oils to calm and soothe headaches. It is also a handy remedy for applying to itchy insect bites and stings.

10 drops peppermint essential oil
5 drops lavender essential oil
5 drops eucalyptus essential oil
10ml (2 teaspoons) carrier oil (page 24)

Mix the essential oils into the carrier oil and pour into an aromatherapy roll-on ball bottle. Label and date.

TO USE Shake gently before each use. Gently roll on as needed around the temples and forehead.

SHELF LIFE Up to 1 year in a cool, dark place.

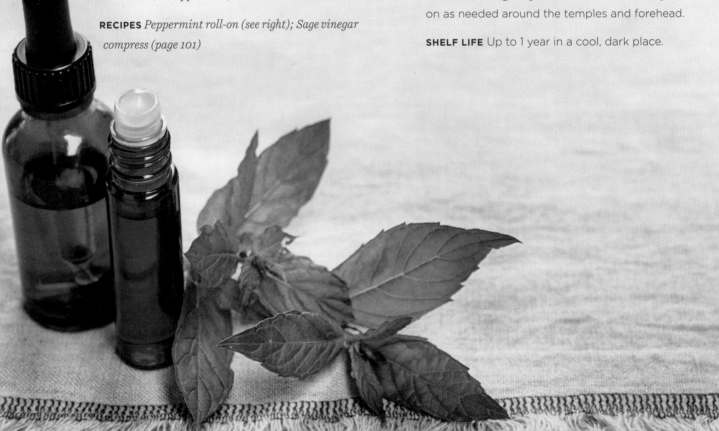

BRUISES

An infused oil or balm of elder leaf, daisy, dandelion flower or St John's wort can be used to clear bruises. Large bruises that affect the head, torso or cover a significant area should be seen by a medical practitioner as there may be a risk of clotting. Constant bruising, or bruises that persist for more than two weeks, should also be seen by a doctor.

INTERNAL HERBS *Hawthorn, yarrow, linden, St John's wort*

EXTERNAL HERBS *Dandelion flower, daisy, elder leaf, St John's wort, horse chestnut leaf or seed, witch hazel, yarrow, arnica, comfrey*

RECIPES *Healing ointment (page 38); Sage vinegar compress (page 101); Comfrey balm (page 104)*

NETTLE STINGS

Nettle sting reactions are usually mild and will quickly disappear. The cooling, anti-inflammatory juice of plantain, chickweed, aloe or nettle can help reduce the inflammation and stinging sensation. Nettle juice can be made by squashing nettle leaves and stems in a plastic bag, ensuring all stings are well crushed, then applying the juice to the affected area.

EXTERNAL HERBS *Nettle, chickweed, aloe vera, plantain*

RECIPES *Chickweed, plantain & aloe poultice (page 40); Skin-soothing gel (page 44); Oaty bath balls (page 129)*

SPLINTERS

Shallow splinters can be removed with a sharp, sterile pin. Apply antiseptic afterwards to prevent infection. If the splinter is deep and reluctant to come out, a simple paste made from water and marshmallow root powder or slippery elm powder, or a fresh plantain leaf poultice can be used overnight to draw it out. Also try the Drawing ointment recipe on page 124.

EXTERNAL HERBS *Marshmallow root, slippery elm, calendula, lavender, witch hazel, plantain, tea tree*

RECIPES *Antimicrobial gel (page 37); Skin-soothing gel (page 44); Drawing ointment (page 124)*

TRAVEL SICKNESS

A condition brought on by motion, causing nausea and/or vomiting. Peppermint, chamomile, ginger and lemon tea can help reduce all sorts of nausea and settle the tummy, or try the recipes suggested below. Apply the Peppermint roll-on to the wrist pulse point. The Happy mummy spray contains essential oils to help with sickness and can be used as a travel spray, too.

INTERNAL HERBS *Ginger, peppermint, chamomile, lemon*

RECIPES *Peppermint roll-on (see opposite); Crystallised ginger & lemon (page 159); Happy mummy spray (page 164)*

BURNS

For minor burns, run the affected area under cold water for at least 20 minutes or until the heat has dispersed. A couple of drops of lavender oil can be applied neat to help with pain and healing in adults. In sensitive people and children, dilute a quarter teaspoon of aloe vera gel with 5 drops of essential oil and apply to the area. Spray burns with cool distilled witch hazel water to bring down inflammation, support the tissues and encourage healing. For sunburn, use the Skin-soothing gel or the Calendula and aloe after-sun cubes below.

EXTERNAL HERBS *Aloe vera gel, calendula, St John's wort, lavender, witch hazel, eucalyptus, nettle, chamomile, yarrow, plantain*

RECIPES *Chickweed, plantain & aloe poultice (page 40); Skin-soothing gel (see right)*

Skin-soothing gel

Harness the cooling properties of aloe vera and witch hazel water in this cooling gel for burns and sunburn. Calendula and St John's wort oil add skin-healing properties, while lavender essential oil eases pain and inflammation.

50ml (2 fl oz) aloe vera gel
1 teaspoon St John's wort infused oil
1 teaspoon calendula infused oil
1 teaspoon witch hazel water
20 drops lavender essential oil

Place the aloe vera gel in a bowl. Drop by drop, gradually whisk in the infused oils and witch hazel water.

Once well combined, mix in the lavender essential oil. Store in a labelled and dated jar.

TO USE Apply liberally to minor burns and sunburn as needed.

SHELF LIFE Up to 3 months in the fridge.

Calendula & aloe after-sun cubes

These versatile, cooling calendula, aloe and lavender cubes help soothe and take down the inflammation of sunburn, minor burns, insect bites, stings, cuts, bruises and itchy rashes. For external use only.

4 tablespoons fresh calendula petals
100ml (3½ fl oz) boiling water
150ml (5 fl oz) aloe vera gel
1 tablespoon honey
20 drops lavender essential oil

Infuse the calendula petals in the water for 15 minutes. Blend the aloe vera gel, honey and calendula infusion (with the petals) together until smooth. Stir in the lavender essential oil. Pour into ice cube trays and place in the freezer. Once frozen, store in an airtight container in the freezer.

TO USE Rub 1–2 cubes over sore, tender areas.

SHELF LIFE Up to 6 months in the freezer.

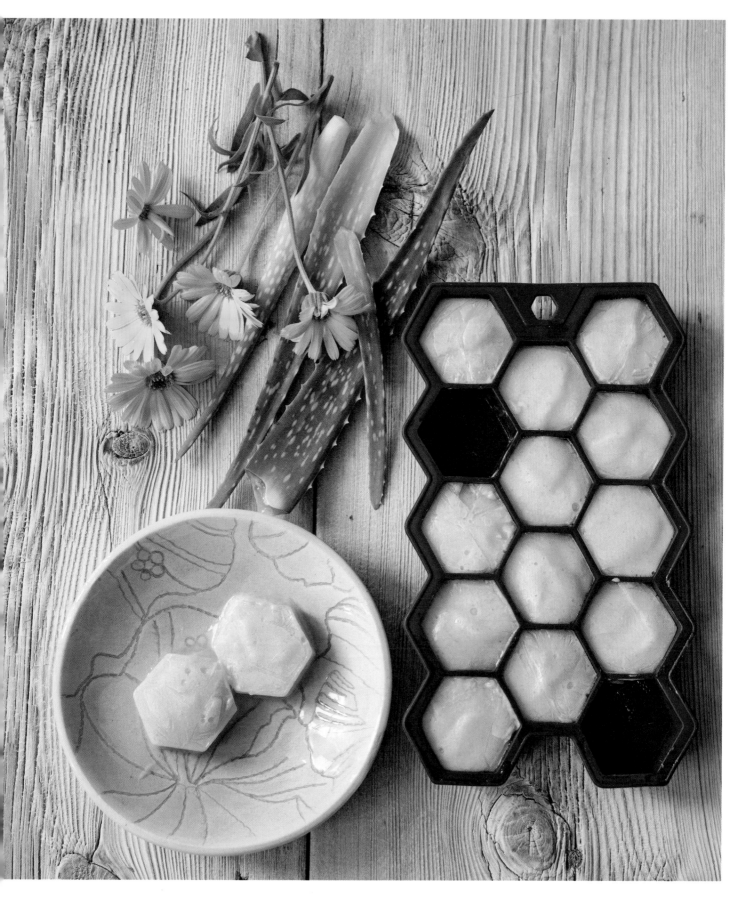

MOUTH ULCERS

These are small, painful blisters found on the mouth and tongue, usually caused by damage to the tissues from abrasions, nutritional deficiencies or a reaction to certain foods. Some people are prone to idiopathic (spontaneous) blisters with no obvious cause, and women tend to suffer from mouth ulcers more commonly than men. Toning, anti-inflammatory herbal gargles can help to heal and soothe painful ulcers containing calendula or blackberry leaf. Keep foods that are high in B12, zinc and iron plentiful in the diet. Use a healing herbal mouthwash made from strong infusions or diluted tinctures (1 teaspoon of tincture to 30ml/1 fl oz water) from the herbs below, or use the Sore throat gargle recipe on page 119 as a mouthwash.

INTERNAL HERBS *Echinacea, burdock, cleavers, calendula, plantain*

EXTERNAL HERBS *Calendula, thyme, sage, blackberry leaf, echinacea, chamomile, plantain, propolis, myrrh*

RECIPES *Bramble-stop tea (page 72); Sore throat gargle (page 119)*

Mouth ulcer paste

These antiseptic, numbing and healing tinctures are combined with slippery elm or marshmallow root powder to create a paste that can be applied to ulcers as needed. You can buy these tinctures from a good herbal supplier.

2 teaspoons slippery elm or marshmallow root powder
½ teaspoon propolis tincture
½ teaspoon clove tincture
½ teaspoon myrrh tincture
1 teaspoon water

Place the powder in a bowl and add the tinctures and water and mix well. Transfer into a labelled and dated jar.

TO USE Apply a pea-sized blob of this paste to mouth ulcers up to 3 times a day. As the tinctures infuse into the powder, the paste may become thicker, in which case add a few drops of water to work it into a useable consistency.

SHELF LIFE Will keep in an airtight container for up to 1 week in the fridge.

TOOTHACHE

STYES

Toothache can indicate an infection or tooth decay and will need to be seen by a dentist, particularly if the pain recurs or is severe. Tooth enamel cannot be renewed, so good dental hygiene is the most important preventative for dental issues. One drop of clove essential oil, which contains natural anaesthetic eugenol, can be applied with the end of a cotton bud to the area to help temporarily reduce pain (in adults only); clove oil is not to be used long term, however, and you must see a dentist for ongoing pain or infected tooth problems. Support the immune system to help fight infection using echinacea and elderberry tinctures internally. Or try a mouthwash made with the infusion or diluted tinctures of a mixture of echinacea and any of the other herbs below (1 teaspoon of tincture to 30ml/1 fl oz of water).

EXTERNAL HERBS *Echinacea, clove, calendula, thyme, sage, blackberry leaf, plantain, propolis, myrrh*

RECIPES *Sore throat gargle (page 119)*

Styes are caused by a bacterial infection of an oil gland on the eyelid that creates small painful lumps, sometimes filled with pus like a pimple. Bathe the eye with a herbal compress every 4–8 hours, using an infusion of any of the herbs below: soak a piece of cotton in the mixture, leave the pad in place as an eye mask for 5–10 minutes, then gently cleanse the eye.

INTERNAL HERBS *Chamomile, eyebright, plantain, elderflower, white tea, green tea, calendula, yarrow, witch hazel*

RECIPES *Itchy-eye cooler cubes (page 118)*

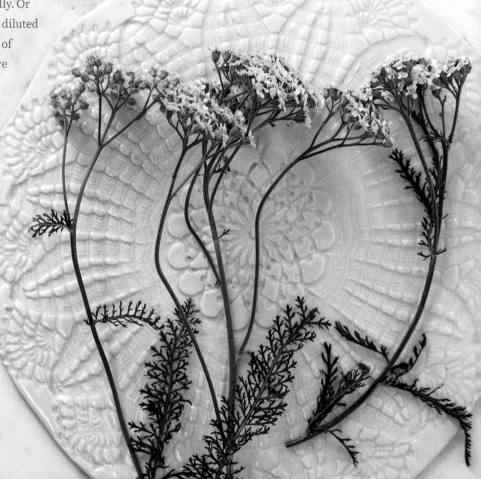

HANGOVER
See page 73.

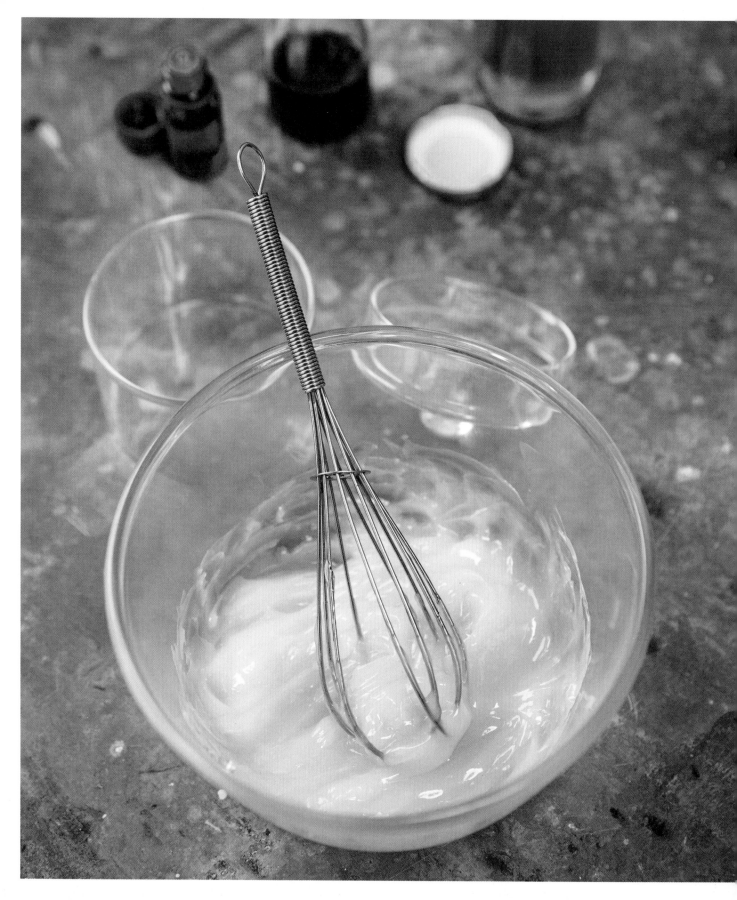

ESSENTIAL OIL RECIPE GUIDE

A quick guide to a handful of recipes using ten staple essential oils. Make these blends for massage or skin application using the guidance box – see right.

INSECT-REPELLENT MIX

Eucalyptus

Lavender

Tea tree

Maximum 5 drops clove

APPLICATIONS

Spray, massage oil, cream, balm

ACHING-MUSCLE MIX

Eucalyptus

Lavender

Rosemary

Frankincense

APPLICATIONS

Massage oil, balm, bath

ANTIFUNGAL MIX

Thyme

Tea tree

Eucalyptus

Maximum 5 drops clove

APPLICATIONS

Cream, spray, powder

ANTISEPTIC MIX

Thyme

Rosemary

Lavender

APPLICATIONS

Cream, spray

HEADACHE MIX

Peppermint

Eucalyptus

Lavender

APPLICATIONS

Temple massage oil or balm

CONGESTION MIX

Eucalyptus or tea tree

Rosemary or thyme

Peppermint

Frankincense

APPLICATIONS

Steam inhalation, bath, chest and back massage oil or balm

MOOD MIX

Frankincense

Geranium

Lavender

APPLICATIONS

Spray, massage oil, bath, room diffuser

SKIN INFECTION/ INFLAMMATION

Yarrow

Lavender

Thyme

Tea tree

APPLICATIONS

Spray, cream, bath

Essential oils are very concentrated volatile oil extracts of aromatic plants. They have general antiseptic properties. because they are so concentrated and have a reasonable shelf like they make great travel remedies and quick remedies to have around the home for first aid purposes. For further explanation about the difference between essential oils and other types of oils see page 24.

USING ESSENTIAL OILS SAFELY

- Essential oils are potent extracts of plant oils. They should be treated with respect and in most cases should not be applied neat to the body.
- Avoid contact with delicate areas such as eyes, ears, nose and genital area.
- Do not take essential oils internally.
- Ensure you buy true essential oils extracted from plants. Some shops sell synthetic fragrance oils these are not essential oils and are toxic.
- When adding essential oils to a bath, ensure you allow it to disperse through the water by first diluting with a carrier oil, bath salts or in a little alcohol, such as vodka, before adding the mixture to the bath. If you do not do this, the essential oil will sit on top of the water, coating the skin as the body enters the water. This can lead to redness, burns and contact dermatitis.

ESSENTIAL OILS RECIPE GUIDE

- **IN CARRIER OILS, BALMS, OINTMENTS AND CREAMS** For every 100ml (3½ fl oz) carrier oil or cream, add 1–3 ml (20–60 drops) of essential oil. A balm can be made by following the instructions on page 26.
- **FOR BATHS** Dilute 4–6 drops of essential oil diluted in 1 teaspoon carrier oil.
- **FOR SPRAY BOTTLES** Add 20–40 drops essential oil to 20ml (4 teaspoons) vodka in a 100ml (3½ fl oz) spray bottle, shake well and then top up with distilled water. This can be used sparingly on the skin and as a room spray. Shake well before use.
- **STEAM INHALATIONS** Use a large bowl that can hold at least 2 litres (3½ pints) of steaming hot water and add 5–10 drops of essential oil. Lean over the bowl, and use a towel to create a 'tent' over the head to capture the steam, which can then be inhaled.

ESSENTIAL OIL	USE
Lavender (*Lavandula* spp.)	**MINOR BURNS** – helps to numb pain and reduce scarring. For adults and children over 12, use 1–2 drops, neat, on affected area. For children younger than 12, dilute 5 drops in 1 teaspoon of essential oil. **SKIN INFECTIONS** – add to base creams to prevent and treat minor skin infections. **SLEEP** – add a few drops to a handkerchief and place by the pillow to aid restful sleep.
Peppermint (*Mentha × piperita*)	**HEADACHES** – dilute 1–5 drops in ½ teaspoon carrier oil and apply to the forehead and temples to ease pain and tension. **BLOATING AND INDIGESTION** – dilute in a carrier oil and massage over the tummy to ease discomfort and flatulence.
Eucalyptus (*Eucalyptus* spp.)	**CONGESTION, COLDS AND FLU** – use in a herbal steam inhalation or add to carrier oils and balms to rub over the chest. **ANTIFUNGAL** – for infected toenails, paint a couple of drops onto the nail twice daily using a cotton bud. For other conditions such as ringworm, athlete's foot and jock itch, add to a base cream and apply to the affected area. Alternatively, a drying powder can be made by combining 5 drops of essential oil with 1 tablespoon arrowroot powder. **COLD SORES** – *Eucalyptus radiata* can be added to lip balms for treating the symptoms of cold sores. **INSECT REPELLENT** – dilute in oil or cream and apply to exposed skin, or use in a spray bottle to deter insects. **MUSCLE PAIN** – dilute eucalyptus oil in a carrier oil and use as a massage oil to ease sore muscles and joints.
Geranium (*Pelargonium graveolens*)	**MOOD** – uplifting to the senses. Dilute in a carrier oil and use as a massage oil or add to a spray bottle and use as a room and pillow spray.

Frankincense (*Boswellia sacra*)	**ASTHMA, CONGESTION** – a few drops added to a room diffuser can encourage deep breathing, supporting asthma sufferers and reducing congestion.
	SKINCARE – frankincense has long been used in skin-healing creams and lotions, where it can improve scarring and reduce the appearance of fine lines and wrinkles.
Thyme (*Thymus vulgaris*)	**ANTIMICROBIAL** – a potent antibacterial and antifungal oil, which can be added to base creams for use on small infected cuts, or for fungal infections, such as ringworm or athlete's foot. Use the lower amount of essential oil drops recommended as this oil is very powerful.
Tea tree (*Melaleuca alternifolia*)	Use in the same way as eucalyptus.
Rosemary (*Rosmarinus officinalis*)	**ANTIMICROBIAL** – dilute in a carrier oil or cream for an anti-infective remedy for cuts and wounds.
	CIRCULATORY STIMULANT – add to creams to improve circulation in the legs and hands.
	HAIR GROWTH AND CONDITIONING – stimulates the circulation to the scalp, helping improve hair growth and quality. Add a couple of drops to your palm-sized squirt of shampoo, or add to carrier oils to make a hair mask (page 137).
	MEMORY STIMULANT – smelling rosemary oil or making a diluted carrier oil for use on pulse points, has been used to improve memory.
Yarrow (*Achillea millefolium*)	**SKIN INFECTION/INFLAMMATION** – antimicrobial and anti-inflammatory for cuts, wounds, eczema, rashes, insect bites and stings. Add to creams, ointments, balms and washes.
Clove (*Syzygium aromaticum*)	**TOOTHACHE** – clove essential oil contains an anaesthetic called eugenol, which helps to temporarily numb pain. Apply a couple of drops to the end of a cotton bud and apply to the sore area only.

CONDITIONS
AROUND THE BODY

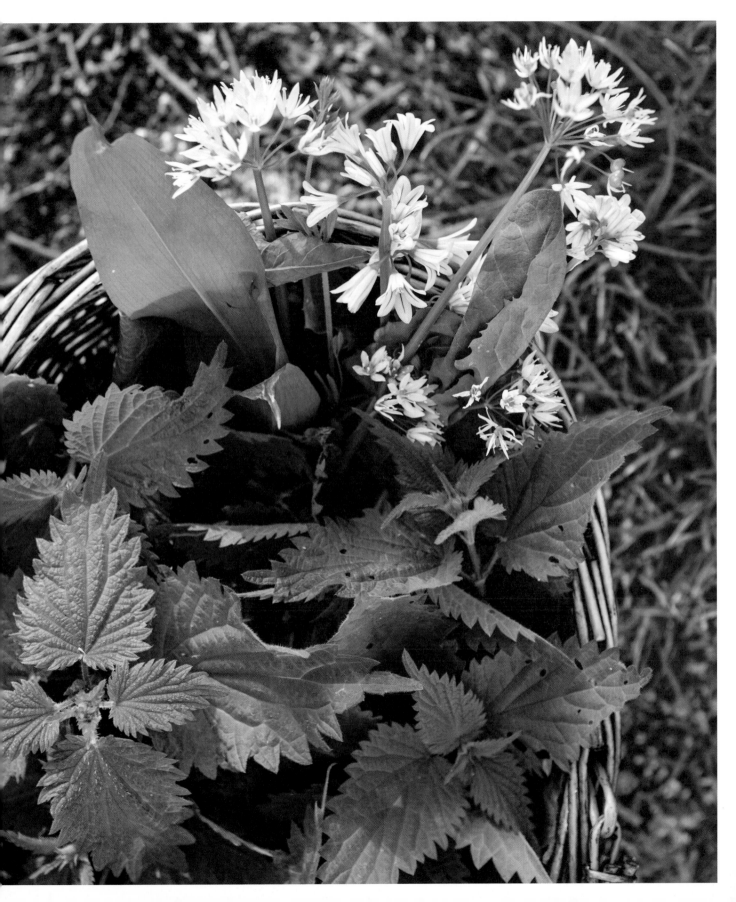

CIRCULATORY HEALTH
ANAEMIA

Simple iron-deficiency anaemia is the reduced ability of the blood cells to carry oxygen around the body, leading to a range of symptoms including fatigue, faintness, headaches, paleness, breathlessness and palpitations. The most common causes of this type of anaemia are low absorption of dietary iron and insufficient red blood cells, usually through blood loss. It can particularly affect menstruating women, especially if flow is heavy.

Increase iron-rich foods in the diet, such as red meats and liver, dark green leafy vegetables and herbs, beetroot, beans and nuts. Vitamin C and B complex help the body absorb iron and form blood cells, and a deficiency in these may require supplementation. Iron absorption can also be inhibited by high intake of tea and coffee. Reduce your consumption, and avoid drinking these within an hour of eating. Drink long/overnight infusions (page 12) of mineral-rich herbs such as nettle, oatstraw and raspberry leaf.

INTERNAL HERBS *Nettle, raspberry leaf, dandelion root and leaf, liquorice, yellow dock, burdock, thyme, sage, marjoram*

RECIPES *Nettle iron drops (page 56); Nettle soup (see right); Nettle & mushroom concentrate powder (page 103); Mineral-rich overnight infusion (page 152); Dark and moody truffles (page 154)*

Nettle soup

Young nettles are rich in circulatory-, tissue- and bone-supporting minerals, including iron, calcium, potassium and zinc. Because of their high protein content, vegetarians and vegans will benefit from adding nettles to their diet.

2 garlic cloves
2 tablespoons cooking oil
1 onion, chopped
150g (5½ oz) mushrooms (any culinary type), chopped (optional)
3 medium potatoes, chopped (peeled if preferred)
1 litre (1¾ pint) hot vegetable stock
1 colander fresh nettle tops
salt and pepper
wild garlic or chive flowers, to garnish (optional)

SERVES 4

Chop the garlic and set aside. (This allows the allicin, one of the main medicinal compounds of garlic, to develop fully.) Heat the oil in a heavy bottomed pan over a medium heat, then add the onion and cook gently until translucent, but not caramelised/browned. Add the mushrooms, if using, and continue to cook until a little soft. Add the chopped potatoes and hot stock to cover. Simmer gently for 15 minutes until the potatoes are cooked.

Add the nettle tops and chopped garlic and continue to simmer gently for a few minutes until the nettles have wilted.

Use a hand blender to blend the soup to a smooth consistency. Season with salt and freshly ground black pepper to taste, and serve with crusty bread.

SHELF LIFE Store in the fridge and use within 3 days. Alternatively, freeze in batches in airtight containers for up to 2 months.

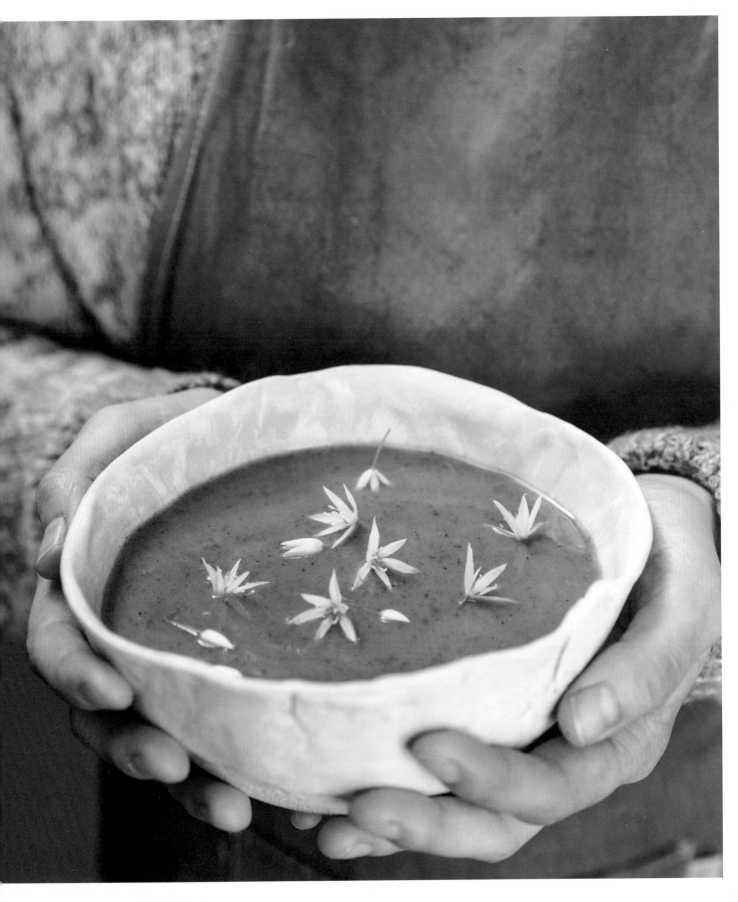

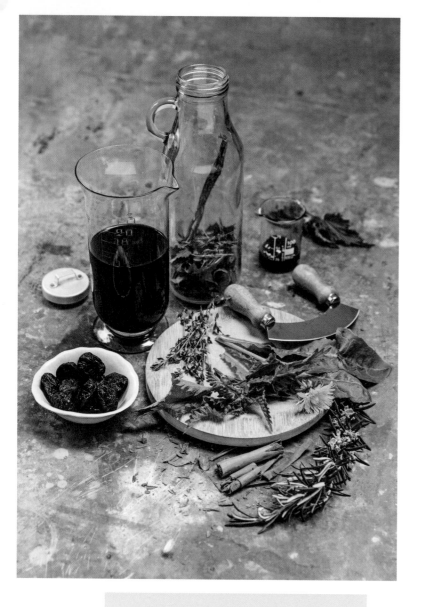

Nettle iron drops

This recipe contains a range of nourishing herbs with a high iron content. Combining different sources of iron is a good way to improve absorption and will add a nutritional spectrum of phytochemicals, minerals and vitamins that aid in healthy circulation and cells.

50g (1¾ oz) fresh nettles

25g (1oz) fresh dandelion leaves

1 tablespoon fresh or dried thyme

1 tablespoon chopped fresh or dried sage

1 tablespoon chopped fresh or dried marjoram

25g (1oz) morel mushrooms (optional)

2 tablespoons fresh or dried yellow dock
   (optional: can make remedy very bitter)

25g (1oz) powdered liquorice

4 tablespoons prunes, apricots, raisins or
   bilberries (or a mix)

2 tablespoons molasses

500ml (18 fl oz) red wine

50ml (2 fl oz) brandy or vodka

Chop the ingredients well (use gloves for the nettles). Place all the ingredients except the wine and brandy in a wide-mouthed jar, then add the red wine and brandy to cover. Close the lid and shake well.

Label and date the jar, then keep in a cool, dark place, shaking gently daily for a month. Strain, discard the solids and retain the liquid in a dark glass bottle.

TO USE Take 1 teaspoon in a little water before food.

SHELF LIFE Up to 1 year in a cool, dark place.

TIPS FOR GATHERING NETTLE TOPS

During spring, gather fresh nettle tops (the youngest top 4–6 leaves) before the plants have gone to flower. After they flower, the leaves become inedible. In autumn, any nettles that have been previously cut back will have a second 'flush' of growth, which can be gathered before they flower again. Use gloves and scissors to snip the tops to avoid stings. Nettles can be dried and crushed (be careful of stings even when dried!) for use all year round.

COLD HANDS, FEET AND CHILBLAINS

Poor circulation to the extremities can result in cold hands and feet, chilblains, palpitations and cramp. It can be aggravated by poor exercise, smoking, poor diet and stress. Herbs that support the circulatory system can be used as infusions or tinctures. Warming herbs and spices, such as rosemary, chilli and ginger can also be made into infused oils and balms. For chilblains, balms using healing herbs such as calendula, comfrey and yarrow help support the capillaries, healing the skin and small wounds.

INTERNAL HERBS *Calendula, rosemary, ginger, cinnamon, hawthorn, linden flower, yarrow, elderflower, cayenne*

EXTERNAL HERBS *Comfrey, calendula, yarrow, gotu kola, rosemary, mustard, ginger, chilli*

RECIPES *Nettle soup (page 54); Warming hand & foot bath (see right); Circulation tonic tea (page 58); Horse chestnut & yarrow leg balm (page 61); Fire cider (page 82); Chilli & ginger joint rub (page 96)*

Warming hand & foot bath

Ideal for cold days and aching feet, or try it as a traditional cold and flu remedy: soak the feet then head to bed for a deep sleep and healing rest.

4 tablespoons mustard seeds (or powder)
4 tablespoons chopped fresh or dried rosemary
5 litres (8¾ pints) boiling water
300g (10½ oz) of Epsom or sea salts

Grind the mustard seeds using a pestle and mortar (or use mustard powder).

Combine the resulting powder with the rosemary and water in a large pan and simmer gently, covered, for 10 minutes.

Allow to cool until it is a suitable temperature for bathing the feet. Add the salts, then pour into a foot bath or bowl.

TO USE Place the foot bath or bowl on a towel. Sit and soak the feet or hands for 15–20 minutes, then remove and dry, massaging gently.

BLOOD PRESSURE

Hawthorn is a specific tonic herb for circulatory issues and is used by herbalists to increase the efficiency of the heart to balance both mild to moderate low and high blood pressure. Dietary and lifestyle choices are vital for a healthy circulatory system, so reduce smoking and consumption of caffeine, alcohol and processed foods high in unsaturated fats and added sugars. Increase fibre and saturated fats, including omega-3s from nuts and oily fish. Garlic, turmeric and beetroot are beneficial for healthy blood vessels and can also be increased in the diet to support good circulatory health.

INTERNAL HERBS *Hawthorn, yarrow, linden flower, rose, motherwort, turmeric, garlic, dandelion*

RECIPES *Nettle soup (page 54); Circulation tonic tea (see right)*

Circulation tonic tea

Hawthorn, the herbalist's specific herb for supporting the heart and circulation, contains oligomeric procyanidins (OPCs) and other flavonoids which are anti-inflammatory, increase circulatory efficiency and help with blood vessel wall integrity. Yarrow, linden and motherwort are also circulatory tonic herbs, with anti-inflammatory effects. This infusion is ideal for all sorts of mild to moderate circulatory issues, palpitations and anxiety.

20g (½ oz) dried hawthorn flowers
20g (½ oz) dried hawthorn berries
20g (½ oz) dried yarrow leaf and flowers
20g (½ oz) dried linden flowers
20g (½ oz) dried motherwort

Mix all the dried herbs together and store in an airtight container.

TO USE Stir 1–2 teaspoons in 200ml (⅓ pint) boiling water. Cover and allow to infuse for 10–15 minutes. Drink up to 3 times a day.

SHELF LIFE Up to 1 year in an airtight container stored in a cool, dark place.

CRAMP
See pages 96–100).

HIGH CHOLESTEROL

VARICOSE VEINS AND HAEMORRHOIDS

There are two main types of cholesterol: low- and high-density lipoproteins (LDL and HDL). A high level of the former is associated with increased risk of heart attacks. The latter (HDL) helps keep the arteries flexible and is beneficial for heart health. Dietary changes are an important approach to reducing 'unfriendly cholesterol'. Increase fibre-rich foods such as fruit and vegetables to help with the body's natural removal of these compounds. Reduce intake of processed foods high in saturated fats, e.g. fatty meats, butter, cheese and cream, and replace with foods containing unsaturated fats, particularly omega-3s, e.g. oily fish, nuts, seeds and avocados. Increasing turmeric and garlic in the diet can also reduce cholesterol levels. Antioxidant herbs taken in infusions or tinctures can help reduce cholesterol levels and improve circulatory health, while red rice yeast supplements have research to support their use in reducing cholesterol.

INTERNAL HERBS *Hawthorn, linden flower, yarrow, elderflower, bilberry, ginger, turmeric, garlic, cinnamon*

RECIPES *Circulation tonic tea (opposite)*

Dilation, swelling and sagging of the veins, particularly in the legs and groin, can cause an aching, heavy feeling. Haemorrhoids are varicose veins of the rectum. Hereditary factors influence the likelihood of developing them, though they can be exacerbated by excessive standing or sitting, constipation, stress and pregnancy. If you have a job that involves sitting or standing, ensure you take regular breaks and try some simple yoga stretches. If constipation is a problem, try the constipation advice on page 62. Try the Circulation tonic tea opposite to support healthy circulation, as well as increasing foods that encourage vein strength, e.g. dark blue and purple foods such as bilberries and elderberries, and rutin-rich foods such as buckwheat and elderflower.

INTERNAL HERBS *Elderflower, elderberry, hawthorn, yarrow, linden flower, bilberry*

EXTERNAL HERBS *Horse chestnut seed and leaf, yarrow, oak bark, witch hazel, elder leaf*

RECIPES *Circulation tonic tea (opposite); Cooling leg spray and Horse chestnut & yarrow balm (page 61)*

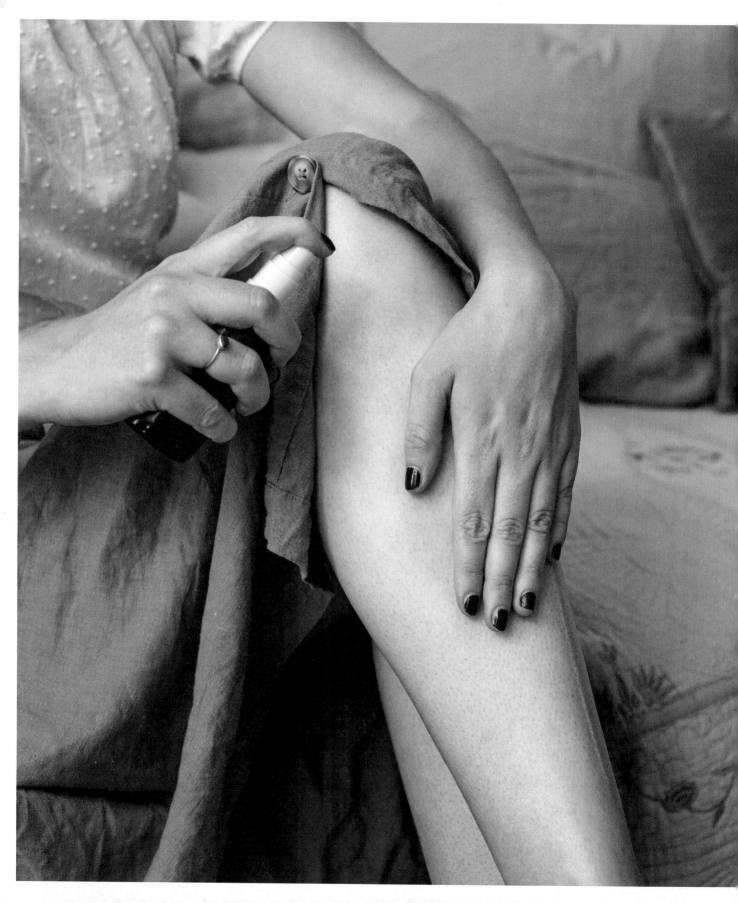

Cooling leg spray

This refreshing spray is ideal for cooling hot, heavy legs on sweltering summer days. It will ease the aches and pains of varicose veins and tone and tighten the skin.

50ml (2 fl oz) witch hazel water

15ml (½ fl oz) aloe vera gel

20ml (4 teaspoons) fresh horse chestnut seed (conker) or leaf tincture

20ml (4 teaspoons) plantain tincture

10ml (2 teaspoons) yarrow infused oil

10 drops cypress essential oil

10 drops rosemary essential oil

Combine all the ingredients in a spray bottle. For best results, store in the fridge to add an extra cooling element.

TO USE Shake the bottle well and spray directly onto legs, massaging gently until absorbed.

SHELF LIFE Up to 6 months in the fridge.

Horse chestnut & yarrow balm

Horse chestnut and yarrow are combined for vein-strengthening properties, and this balm can be used for varicose veins, spider veins, haemorrhoids and leg cramps.

2 teaspoons beeswax

25ml (1 fl oz) horse chestnut leaf and/or seed (conker) infused oil

25ml (1 fl oz) yarrow infused oil

10 drops rosemary essential oil

10 drops cypress essential oil

Using a bain-marie (page 24), gently melt the beeswax into the infused oils. Once completely combined, take off the heat and pour into a 50ml (2 fl oz) jar.

Add the essential oils and stir with a knitting needle or plastic chopstick. Place the lid on and allow to set. Label, date and store in a cool, dark place.

TO USE Massage gently into the legs twice a day.

SHELF LIFE Up to 1 year in a cool, dark place.

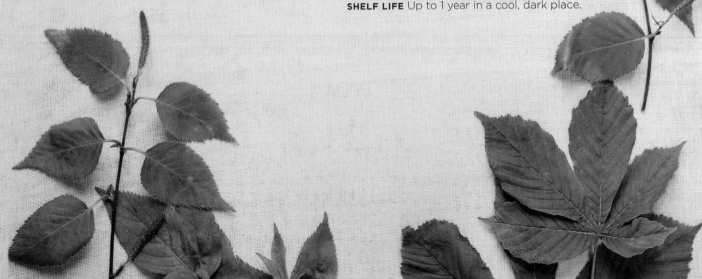

DIGESTIVE HEALTH
BAD BREATH

CONSTIPATION

The most common cause of halitosis, or bad breath, is poor oral hygiene. Ensure you brush your teeth thoroughly after meals to remove any food that may be stuck in between the teeth. If you suffer from persistent bad breath, ensure gum disease is not a cause. Regular trips to the dentist, especially if you notice blood when brushing, will help catch gum disease early. Certain foods can cause bad breath, particularly garlic. This is because the 'garlicky' compound in garlic, allyl methyl sulfide, is carried in the bloodstream, breaks down slowly over a few hours and diffuses out of the lungs. Chewing a sprig of parsley or mint after meals may help freshen breath temporarily.

Another factor involved in bad breath is poor digestion. If food is slow to pass through the digestive system, the processes involved in food breakdown are more likely to produce gases and smells that can pass 'up' as well as 'down'. Investigate digestive issues such as constipation, poor gut flora and upset digestion, and also any food sensitivities which may need to be reviewed by a healthcare professional. For a quick fix, chew a few herbs from the following list.

INTERNAL HERBS *Cardamom seed, fennel seed, caraway, yarrow, peppermint, dandelion, curly dock, burdock, mahonia*

RECIPES *Bitter digestive spray (page 66); Fennel & mint after-dinner pyramids (page 69); Ashwagandha, flax & chia seed pudding (page 152)*

Constipation symptoms include passing faeces less than three times in a week, and stools that are difficult to pass or are uncomfortable, dry or hard. Causes can include a lack of fluids, lack of dietary fibre, tension and anxiety, lack of exercise and some types of medicine. Occasional constipation can be relieved by increasing fluid intake, or fibre intake (from fruit, vegetables, or cereals such as oats). Prune juice is a simple and effective remedy that is available from most shops. Herbal supplements for constipation include the use of bitters, such as dandelion or dock root decoction, or tincture (page 14), which stimulate the liver to produce bile, the body's natural laxative. Bulk-forming laxatives using gloopy seeds such as chia seed, flax seed or psyllium husk help to 'moisten' and 'bulk' out stools, making them easier to pass. The use of harsh 'irritant laxatives' such as senna pods or cascara should be used only in extreme circumstances, and should not be used regularly as the body can come to rely on them. If you suffer from constipation regularly, haven't passed a stool for more than a few days and are not improving with treatment, particularly in the very young or elderly, seek advice from your doctor.

INTERNAL HERBS *Dandelion root, curly dock, mahonia, flax seed, chia seed, psyllium husk, liquorice*

RECIPES *Psyllium gel and Fig & prune syrup (see opposite); Bitter digestive spray (page 66)*

Fig & prune syrup

This tasty syrup contains figs and prunes, which have a gentle laxative effect. With the softening and bulking properties of sugar, this sweet, beautiful ruby-red syrup should help ease things along.

150g (5½ oz) or approximately 4 fresh figs
150g (5½ oz) or approximately 4 dried prunes
450ml (16 fl oz) water
at least 300g (10½ oz) sugar or 300ml (½ pint)
   date syrup
1 teaspoon citric acid or juice of 1 lemon

Place the figs, prunes and the water (or just enough to cover the ingredients) in a pan. Gently simmer for 20–30 minutes, until the fruit starts to break down and become mushy.

Remove the mixture from the heat and allow to sit, covered, until cool enough to handle. Strain out the fruit pulp by passing it through a muslin-lined sieve. Measure your strained liquid and return to the pan. For every 100ml (3½ fl oz)of liquid you have, add 75g (2½ oz) sugar or 75ml (2½ fl oz) date syrup, then simmer gently until the liquid has thickened. Stir in the citric acid or lemon juice.

While still hot, pour into a sterilised jar, label and date.

TO USE Take 2–3 tablespoons, 2–3 times a day. If symptoms persist, seek professional help.

SHELF LIFE Up to 3 months in the fridge.

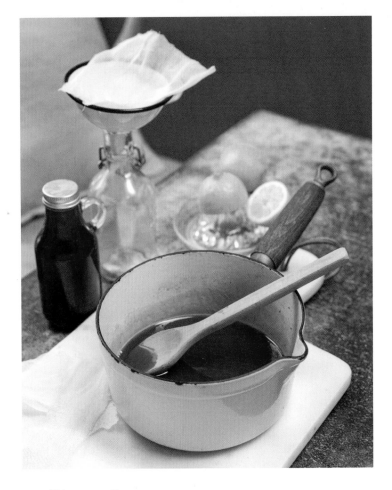

Psyllium gel

A soothing gel to help ease constipation and digestive inflammation. If taking medication, wait an hour before using as it can prevent absorption.

2 tablespoons dried dandelion root (optional)
300ml (½ pint) water
2 teaspoons psyllium husks

In a pan, gently simmer the dandelion root (if using) in the water for 10–15 minutes, then allow to sit for 10–15 minutes. Strain, discarding the solids and retain the liquid. If you don't have dandelion root, just use the water. In a cup or bowl, place the psyllium and decoction liquid (at least 200ml/⅓ pint). Either drink right away or leave until the husks have created a gel-like consistency, then drink.

TO USE Drink 200ml (⅓ pint) up to 2–3 times a day. If no relief after 48 hours, seek medical advice.

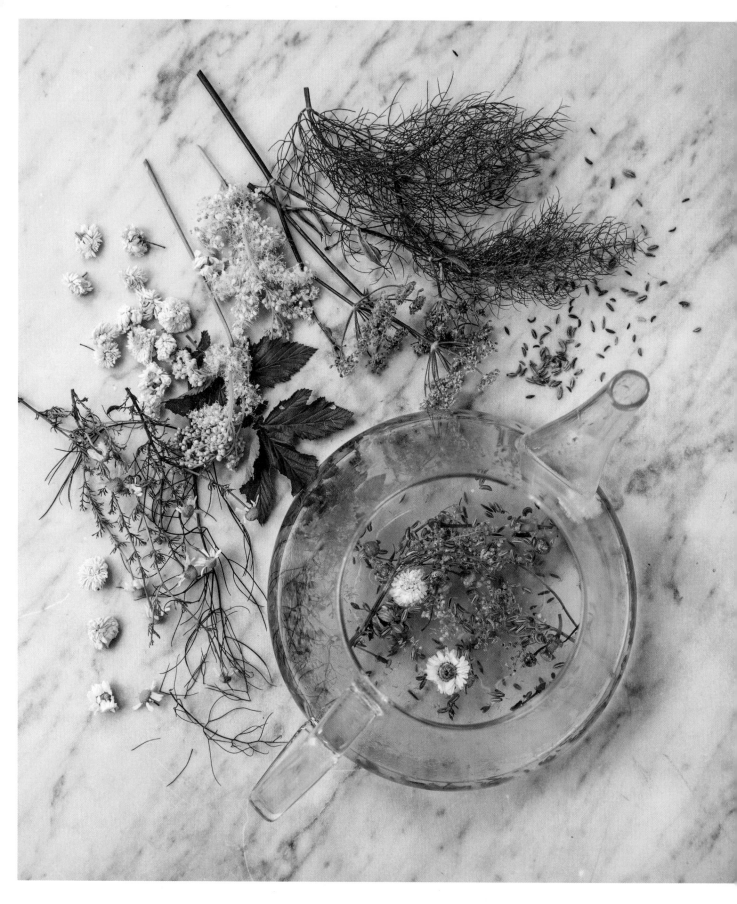

INDIGESTION & HEARTBURN

Occasional uncomfortable digestion can be caused by trapped wind or muscle spasms. Infusions of the herbs below can soothe muscle cramps and disperse gasses. Acid reflux, or heartburn, is the overspill of harsh stomach acid into the lower tube of the oesophagus. This can happen from time to time in healthy individuals and can be caused by overly large or rich meals, too much coffee or alcohol, smoking, pregnancy or a weak sphincter muscle at the top of the stomach (which should 'hold in' the stomach contents). With heartburn, avoid peppermint tea, as mint relaxes the muscles of the digestive system. While this makes it ideal for other types of indigestion and tummy pains, it can increase acid reflux as the sphincter muscle at the top of the stomach will also relax and become more 'leaky'. Chronic indigestion or heartburn may be due to food sensitivities or other underlying conditions and will need to be investigated by your doctor or herbalist.

INTERNAL HERBS *Chamomile, meadowsweet, aniseed, cardamom, fennel, peppermint (not in acid reflux)*

RECIPES *After-dinner tea (see right); Bitter digestive spray (page 66); Fennel and mint after-dinner pyramids (page 69)*

After-dinner tea

This recipe uses a traditional herbal blend that helps reduce and soothe after-dinner acid reflux and indigestion, tummy ache and flatulence.

25g (1oz) chamomile dried flowers
25g (1oz) meadowsweet dried flowers
10g (¼ oz) fennel seeds
200ml (⅓ pint) boiling water

Mix all the ingredients except the water together in a bowl.

TO USE Place a dessertspoon of the mix in a mug and cover with the boiling water. Cover and allow to infuse for 15 minutes. Sip after dinner and repeat as required.

SHELF LIFE Store in an airtight container in a cool, dark place for up to 1 year.

HERBAL BITTERS

Medical herbalists believe that the seat of good health lies in the digestion and will often prescribe bitter herbs when poor digestion is associated with poor health. The traditional 'aperitif' or bitter pre-dinner drink such as gin and tonic is part of the tradition of taking bitters before food to stimulate digestion.

When bitter herbs are tasted on the tongue, a message is sent via the vagus nerve to the brain. This sets off a chain reaction along the whole digestive system, which stimulates the salivary glands, stomach, pancreas and liver to produce digestive juices and enzymes.

These juices help the effective breakdown and absorption of molecules and encourage the removal of waste from the body. Bitter herbs can stimulate a poor appetite and also give a feeling of satisfaction after eating well. They are prescribed for a range of digestive complaints, including poor appetite, heartburn and constipation.

Skin conditions, hormonal issues and some allergies, when associated with digestive problems, can also be helped with bitters. This is because problems such as poor absorption of nutrients, sluggish liver processes and constipation, which delays elimination of waste, can impact the optimal function of the body. During bowel movements, it is not just undigested food that is passed but also spent hormones, dead cells and metabolic waste. Slow and sluggish digestive transition means that these stay in the gut longer than needed, which allows some to be reabsorbed into the bloodstream, putting more pressure on the eliminatory organs such as the liver and skin. However, these can be complex conditions and if they persist, seek guidance from a herbalist.

Bitter digestive spray

SIMPLE BITTERS
dandelion root and/or leaf
burdock root and/or seeds

AROMATIC BITTERS
yarrow flower and leaf
angelica root
juniper berry
mugwort leaf

SOUR BITTERS
fresh ginger root
grapefruit peel
berberis/mahonia berry

ASTRINGENT BITTERS
berberis/mahonia berries or bark
oak bark

OTHER INGREDIENTS
vodka

Take one or more ingredients (they can be fresh or dried) from each of the four groups of bitters above, and chop or grind finely. Loosely fill a 250ml (9 fl oz) jar with the herbs to about three-quarters full and fill to the neck of the jar with vodka. Seal the lid, label and date. Allow to infuse for 1 month, shaking occasionally. Strain the liquid into a dropper or spray bottle, label and date.

TO USE Take 2 sprays, 10 drops or ½ teaspoon 15–30 minutes before food.

CONTRAINDICATIONS Avoid during pregnancy and lactation, for those with stomach ulcers and children under 12 years.

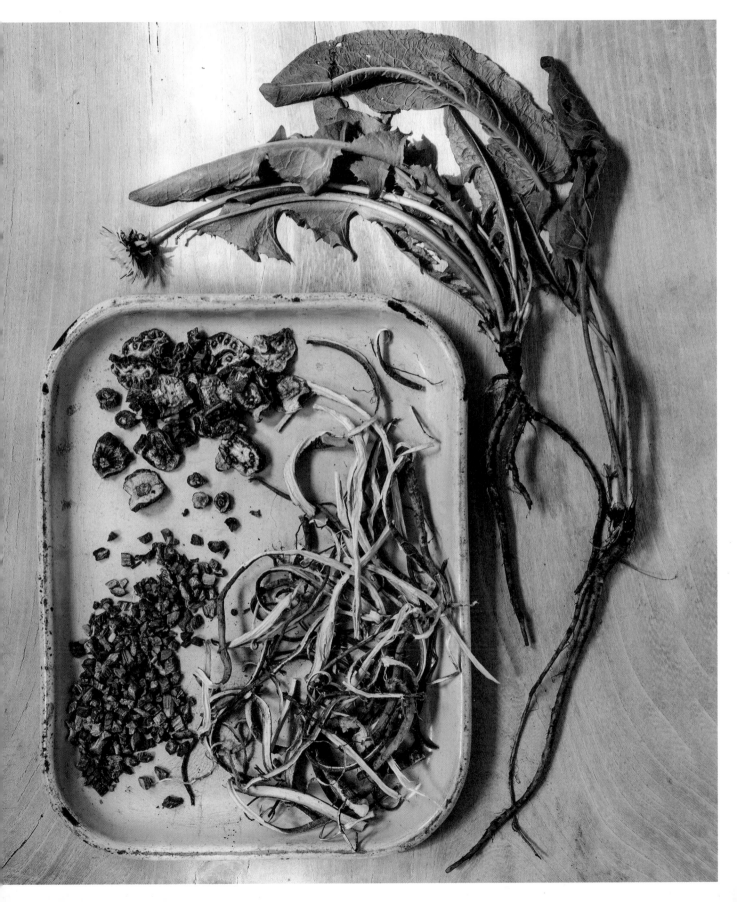

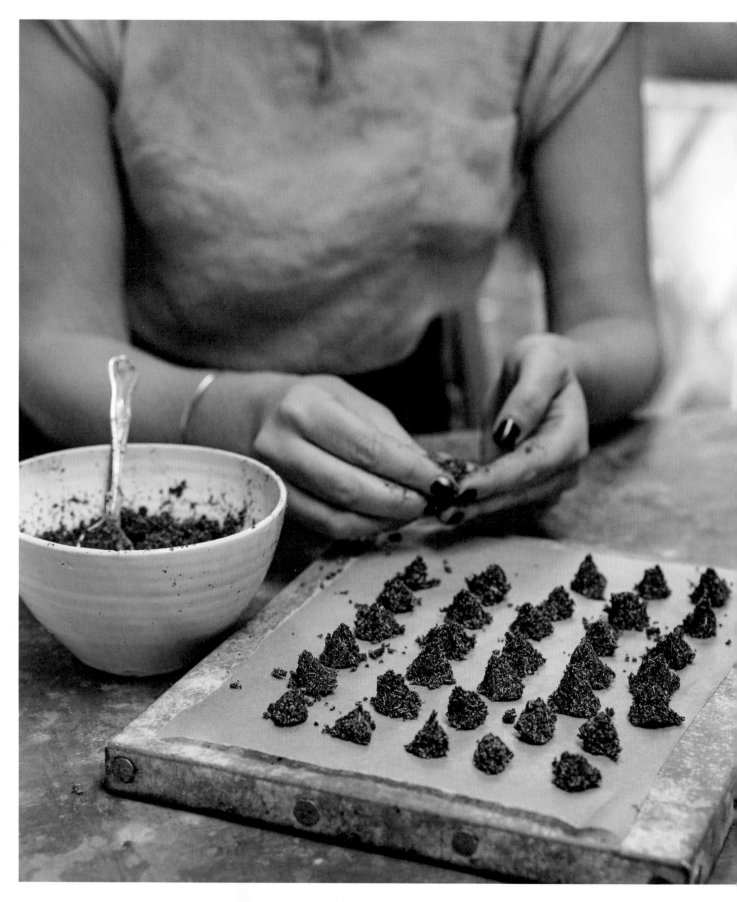

FLATULENCE

To reduce flatulence, make sure you chew your food well, and try to avoid gulping air in a rush to eat as it may cause trapped air and wind. Sometimes the pressure of wind can strain the digestive system, causing spasms and tummy ache. Herbal teas using 'carminative' herbs help soothe spasms, reduce the production of, and dispel, wind. Some foods such as pulses, including beans and peas, give people excessive gas. In Japanese cooking, a piece of seaweed (kombu or wakame) is added while cooking pulses, which makes them more digestible and reduces flatulence. Aromatic spices and herbs added to cooking can also reduce the production of digestive gas. Slow digestion or imbalanced gut flora (page 66) can increase the chances of producing wind, and herbal teas or bitter drops can help improve gut transition time.

INTERNAL HERBS *Fennel seed, aniseed, caraway, cardamom, black pepper, chamomile, ginger, peppermint*

RECIPES *After-dinner tea (page 65); Bitter digestive spray (page 66); Fennel & mint after-dinner pyramids (see right)*

Fennel & mint after-dinner pyramids

These pastilles can be chewed after meals to help prevent and ease stomach upsets and flatulence. If you suffer from acid reflux, replace the mint with chamomile flowers.

10g (¼ oz) fennel seeds
5g (⅛ oz) dried peppermint leaves
5g (⅛ oz) dried meadowsweet flowers
2 teaspoons marshmallow root or slippery elm powder
a little honey (or use glycerine for a vegan option)
a little boiled water

Grind all the dry ingredients to a fine powder using a pestle and mortar or a strong food processor. Place the powder in a bowl and add a little honey and water, a teaspoon at a time, until a smooth paste forms. Take a small pinch of the mixture (about the size of a small marble) and squeeze the paste between your fingers to make a little pyramid or ball. Lay out on baking parchment to dry fully in a warm place, or use a dehydrator.

TO USE After eating, chew one pyramid and wash down with a little water.

SHELF LIFE Up to 3 months in an airtight container in the fridge.

NAUSEA & VOMITING

DIARRHOEA & GASTROENTERITIS

These may be symptoms of stress, poor digestion, over-indulgence, a sensitivity to food or drugs, or motion sickness when travelling. Mild symptoms may be settled with a fresh ginger root tea or crystallised ginger pieces, both of which are safe options for pregnancy-induced nausea, too. Nausea or upset tummy can also be helped by chewing fresh thyme leaves or using some bitter drops to settle the stomach (page 66). For pregnancy-related nausea, see page 159. Seek professional help if you have vomited for more than two days, and are very young or elderly.

INTERNAL HERBS *Ginger, meadowsweet, chamomile, angelica, thyme, fennel, aniseed, peppermint, cardamom*

RECIPES *Bitter digestive spray (page 66); Fennel & mint after-dinner pyramids (page 69); Hangover powders (page 73); Crystallised ginger & lemon (page 159)*

Chronic, long-term diarrhoea could be a sign of an underlying issue such as colitis or diverticulitis, which are complicated issues best addressed by a healthcare practitioner. In bacterial food poisoning, vomiting and diarrhoea are the body's way of removing unwanted toxins, so should only be curbed if excessive or persistent. In these cases, try the astringent Bramble-stop tea (page 72). The use of antimicrobial, antispasmodic and drying 'astringent' herbs helps soothe the digestive system and reduce symptoms of discomfort.

For recovery and restoration of the digestive system after illness, slow cooked bone (or mushroom) broths (pages 76 and 78) with plenty of anti-infective garlic will provide nutrients to restore the inflamed gut lining. Drink plenty of water to maintain hydration and take rehydration salts to restore the body's level of electrolytes.

A basic rehydration salts recipe contains ½ teaspoon of salt and 4 teaspoons of sugar mixed into 500ml (8 fl oz) of warm water. Sip throughout the day. If you are unable to keep fluids down, are bleeding, or have diarrhoea for more than three days, especially in the young, elderly or those who are health-compromised, seek professional help.

INTERNAL HERBS *Chamomile, thyme, garlic, rosemary, sage, lavender, fennel seed, blackberry fruit, bramble leaf, oak bark, willow bark, meadowsweet*

RECIPES *Oral rehydration salts (see opposite); Bramble-stop tea (page 72); Hangover powders (page 73)*

Oral rehydration salts

These rehydration salts help to replace the body's lost minerals through the excessive fluid loss of vomiting and diarrhoea. The thyme and chamomile infusion adds antispasmodic and antimicrobial properties to ease discomfort and to help with combating any bacterial infection.

1 teaspoon fresh or dried thyme
1 teaspoon fresh or dried chamomile flowers
500ml (8 fl oz) boiling water
½ teaspoon salt
4 teaspoons sugar or honey

Chop or grind the thyme and chamomile finely and place in a pan. Pour over the boiling water, cover and leave to infuse until tepid. Strain the liquid and stir in the salt and sugar or honey until dissolved.

If you do not have the herbs to hand, you can make a basic rehydration recipe with the water, sugar and salt dissolved together.

TO USE Sip this liquid throughout the day.

SHELF LIFE Use within 24 hours.

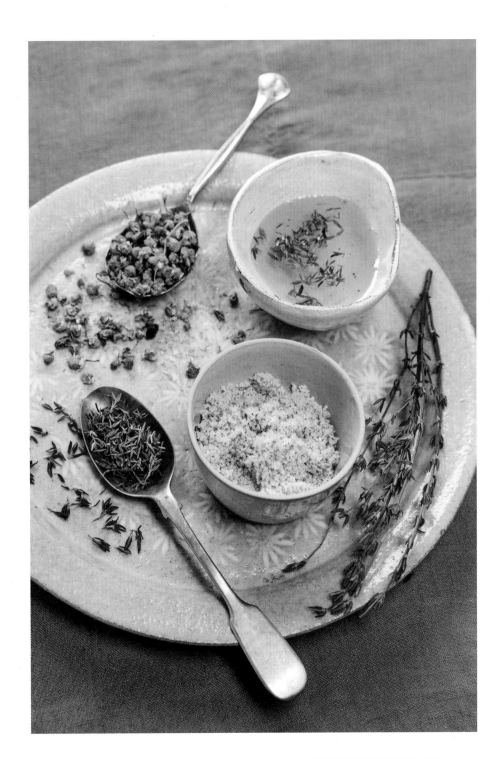

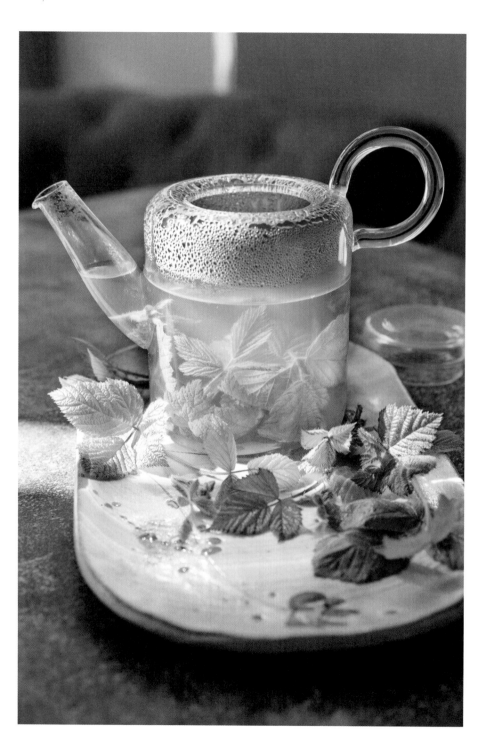

Bramble-stop tea

A simple blackberry leaf tea is an astringent (dries up secretions) infusion that will aid in reducing urgent diarrhoea and help combat urinary tract infections. It can also be used as a gargle to tone sore throats and a mouthwash to help heal mouth ulcers. Gather and dry fresh spring bramble leaves. Nettle leaf and blackberries contain restorative minerals and vitamins, while thyme has an antimicrobial action.

25g (1oz) fresh or dried blackberries (optional)
25g (1oz) fresh or dried blackberry leaves
10g (¼ oz) fresh or dried thyme
10g (¼ oz) fresh or dried nettles
200ml (⅓ pint) boiling water

Mix all the ingredients together, except the water, in a bowl.

TO USE Place a dessertspoon of the mix in a mug and cover with the boiling water. Allow to infuse for 10–15 minutes. Drink up to 3 cups a day in slow, gradual sips.

SHELF LIFE Up to 1 year in an airtight jar in a cool, dark place.

HANGOVER

The dreaded hangover that comes after a night of over-indulgence is not something that generally puts us off over-indulging in the first place! Whether your symptoms are nausea, upset tummy, headache or anxiety, the following hangover powder recipe can help support and protect the liver while it is working extra hard to bring the body back into a state of health. A herbalist's secret is to take a teaspoon of ground milk thistle seeds either in an infusion or in a little honey to help it slip down, before you head out for an evening of indulgence – whether it is lots of food, alcohol or both!

RECIPES *Hangover powders (see right)*

MILK THISTLE

Milk thistle is a go-to hangover herb. Research has shown a constituent called silymarin helps to protect liver cells from damage from toxins from things such as medications and alcohol. The seeds are nutty and slightly bitter. For hangovers, it works best as a preventative, 1 teaspoon can be chewed before you head for a night out!

Hangover powders

This herbal mix contains milk thistle, which has liver-protecting properties and is commonly used by herbalists to help with hangovers. The other bitter herbs, such as the willow, along with ginger and meadowsweet help settle upset tummies. The meadowsweet, turmeric and willow also contain potent anti-inflammatories to soothe inflamed stomach tissue and help to ease aches, pains and headaches. The mucilaginous (gloopy) marshmallow root or slippery elm powder soothes an irritated digestive tract.

1 tablespoon dried milk thistle seeds
1 teaspoon ground ginger
1 tablespoon meadowsweet flowers
1 teaspoon ground turmeric
1 tablespoon marshmallow root or slippery elm powder
1 teaspoon honey or 50ml (2 fl oz) warm water

In a blender, whizz the dried milk thistle seeds to a powder. Add the rest of the dried herbs and pulse in the blender until it becomes a smooth, even powder.

TO USE Stir 1 dessertspoon of the powder into 1 teaspoon of honey or 50ml (2 fl oz) of warm water and leave to stand for 10 minutes. Take before bed and the morning after, and repeat as needed throughout the day.

SHELF LIFE Store in a cool, dark place in an airtight container for up to 6 months.

IMMUNITY & INFECTION
FEVER

Fever is classified as a rise in body temperature above 38°C. It is usually the result of a natural immune response by the body to a foreign invader, commonly a bacteria or virus. In the case of a mild fever, it is widely recommended to let it run its course, the idea being that the fever is doing its job: raising the body temperature to create an inhospitable environment for invaders. If fever becomes uncomfortable, particularly if it is affecting sleep, try drinking an infusion of febrifuge (fever-reducing) herbs, including elderflower, yarrow or chamomile; they encourage sweating and allow dilation of the blood vessels near the surface of the skin to disperse heat. Treat the underlying infection with anti-infective herbs such as elderberry and echinacea, which support the immune system to fight the infection

CAUTION Seek medical attention for a fever of 38°C (100°F) or more in babies under 6 months; for high fever in children and the elderly; or if body temperature reaches 40°C (104°F).

INTERNAL HERBS *Linden flower, elderflower, peppermint, yarrow, chamomile, peppermint, elderberry, echinacea*

RECIPES *Herbal hot toddy (see right); Bone broth (page 76); Mushroom tonic soup (page 77); Vegan mushroom broth (page 78); Immune tincture (page 80)*

Herbal hot toddy

Many old herbals recommend drinking a hot toddy before bed to 'sweat out' a fever. This recipe uses elderflower, which is antiviral and encourages sweating, helping to bring down a temperature, while lemon juice and honey help to soothe a sore throat.

1 tablespoon grated fresh ginger root
1 teaspoon dried elderflowers
5 cloves
1 cinnamon stick, crumbled (optional)
300ml (½ pint) boiling water
½–1 tablespoon honey
25–50ml (1–2 fl oz) brandy, whisky, rum or spiced rum
juice of ½ lemon
1 teaspoon dried linden flowers

Place the grated ginger, elderflower, cloves and cinnamon (if using) in a teapot. Pour over the boiling water, cover and allow this to infuse for 5–10 minutes.

Place the honey, brandy/whisky/rum and lemon juice in a mug and pour over the hot tea through a strainer. Stir well and drink immediately.

SHELF LIFE Suitable for adults only. Drink 1 cup before bed. This recipe is high in alcohol, so do not drive or operate machinery after drinking. Alternatively, for children, omit the alcohol and reduce the dosage, as per instructions on page 138.

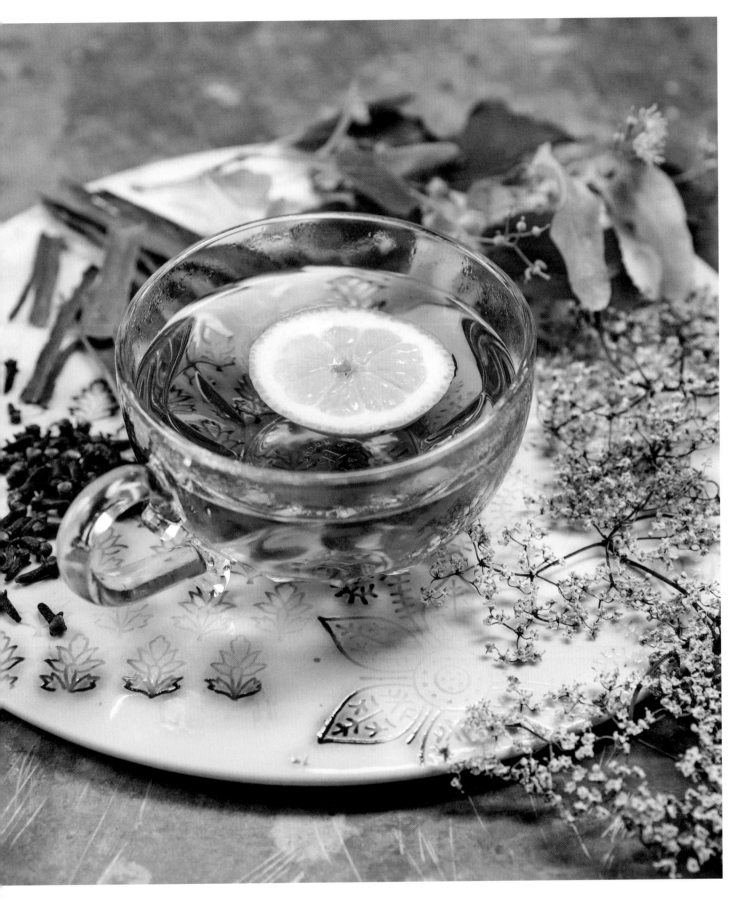

CONVALESCENCE

Convalescence is the period after a trauma or illness during which the body needs to recover. Recovery times after illness can vary hugely, and this is especially true for viral infections. During convalescence, the body, mind and muscles can feel weak and tired, so it is important to have adequate rest, taking time to sleep, relax and nourish the body to restore strength and vitality. Eat vitamin- and mineral-rich foods and teas and plenty of protein to help repair damaged tissues.

Medicinal mushrooms have a balancing effect on the immune system and are particularly helpful when the immune system has been taxed. Eat plenty of shiitake and even plain old button mushrooms in soups and stews during the convalescence period. Ginseng has a long traditional use for increasing stamina and strengthening the body after illness; this is best taken in decoction or tincture form (pages 12–14).

INTERNAL HERBS *Maitake, shiitake, chaga, turkey tail, echinacea, garlic, onions, nettle, ginseng, horsetail, elderberry, oats, oatstraw, ashwagandha, cocoa*

RECIPES *Bone broth (see right); Vegan mushroom broth (page 78); Mushroom tonic soup (see opposite); Immune tincture (page 80); Nettle soup (page 54); Fire cider (page 82)*

Bone broth

Many a grandmother will tell you that chicken soup is a cure for everything! Slow-cooked chicken soup contains a wide range of vitamins, minerals, amino acids and protein helpful for the growth and renewal of tissues, including skin and joints. It is particularly beneficial for gut health and healing. This densely nutritious broth supplies the body with all of the immune-boosting minerals, vitamins and amino acids it needs during times of illness and convalescence.

1 large onion, chopped

2 carrots, sliced

3 celery sticks, chopped

1 raw or cooked organic chicken carcass,
   or 10–15 organic chicken wings

2 handfuls of fresh or 1 handful of dried nettle leaves

4 garlic cloves, crushed

a few sprigs of fresh thyme

½–1 teaspoon freshly crushed black pepper

4 bay leaves

1–2 teaspoons of salt or stock powder concentrate

2 litres (3½ pints) water

Place all of the ingredients in a large saucepan, bring to the boil, then reduce the heat and simmer gently, covered, for 3–4 hours, adding more water if necessary.

Strain off the liquid and reserve. Also reserve the chicken meat for returning to the broth, or for use in other recipes, but discard the remaining solids. Drink this broth alone or add to soups, stews or risottos.

Alternatively, scoop out and discard the chicken bones, bay leaves, thyme stalks and nettle leaves, then blend into a smooth soup using a stick blender.

SHELF LIFE Keep in the fridge for up to 3 days, or in the freezer for up to 6 months.

Mushroom tonic soup

After acute illness, your appetite can suffer. This nourishing 'miso' stock powder can be made in minutes and drunk by the mugful for a quick but powerful nutritional blast. It can also be added to other stocks, sauces and soups for a heartier meal.

1 tablespoon garlic powder

2 tablespoons dried onion flakes

1 tablespoon turkey tail powder

2 teaspoons ground celery seeds

2 tablespoons powdered or crumbled seaweed

2 tablespoons powdered nettle leaves

2–3 teaspoons ground rock salt

1 tablespoon shiitake powder

1 tablespoon chaga powder

spring onion, mushrooms, tofu
   or fresh herbs, to serve

Mix all the dried ingredients together and store in an airtight container in a cool, dark place.

TO USE Add 1 or 2 teaspoons of soup powder to a cup and top up with boiling water. Sprinkle with finely diced spring onion, tofu or other fresh culinary herbs. Drink 1–2 cups a day.

SHELF LIFE The dry powder will keep in an airtight container for up to 6 months.

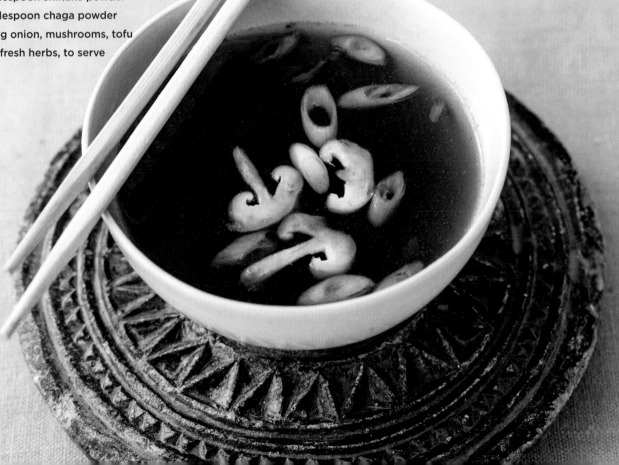

Vegan mushroom broth

This vegan 'bone' broth uses shiitake mushrooms, high in healing minerals such as potassium, magnesium and zinc, as well as immune-boosting beta-glucans. Serves 4.

200g (7oz) shiitake or a mix of other speciality
   mushrooms, such as oyster, enoki and
   maitake, sliced
1 strip of kombu seaweed
30g (1 oz) wakame seaweed
2 handfuls of fresh or 1 handful
   of dried nettle leaves
2 litres (3½ pints) water
1 large onion, chopped
3 large garlic cloves, crushed and sliced
2 carrots, sliced
3 celery sticks, chopped
1–2 tablespoons soy sauce
100g (3½ oz) vermicelli noodles
1 chilli, sliced
lime wedges, to serve
2 spring onions, sliced, to serve
few coriander sprigs, to serve

Place the mushrooms, seaweeds and nettles in a large saucepan and pour over the water. Bring to the boil and then reduce to a gentle simmer, covered, for 1–2 hours, adding more water, if necessary. Strain out the nettle leaves. Add the onion, garlic, carrots, celery sticks and soy sauce and simmer for a further 5-10 minutes. You can then strain the solids out and drink this broth alone or add to soups, stews or risottos. For a tasty noodle soup option, don't strain the vegetables out, add the noodles (cook as per instructions), then garnish with sliced chilli, spring onions, coriander and lime wedges.

SHELF LIFE Keep in the fridge for up to 3 days, or in the freezer for up to 6 months.

MUSHROOMS

All mushrooms contain compounds beneficial to immune health, even the standard white button mushrooms commonly found in supermarkets. However 'medicinal mushrooms' such as reishi, shiitake, chaga and turkey tail also contain contain various polysaccharides including b-glucans and a-glucans (among many others) that are used in medicinal preparations for the immune system, acting as a modulator that boosts the immune system when it is under-active and keeps it in check when it becomes over-active. Mushrooms also contain vitamin D (boost vitamin D in mushrooms by laying them in the sun, gill side up, for an hour before eating or using in medicine). Vitamin D is essential for a healthy functioning immune system, again by having a modulating effect.

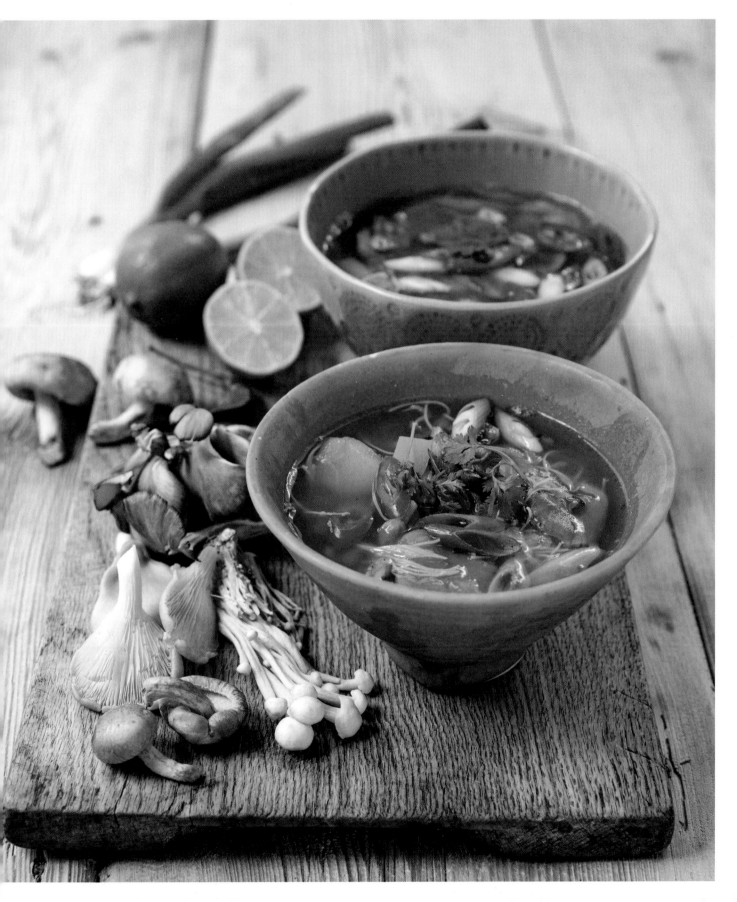

BACTERIAL INFECTIONS

General bacterial infections are best treated herbally by boosting the immune system. The body uses more vitamins, minerals and nutrients when it is fighting infection, in particular vitamins C and B complex, and zinc. For local infections such as an infected cut or chest infection, refer to the section for that ailment, as there are some herbs that have anti-infective actions on specific organs and tissues. Immune-boosting herbs such as echinacea and elderberry can help fight infection, while lymphatic herbs such as cleavers and calendula can aid the body in removing infection.

INTERNAL HERBS *Garlic, echinacea, onion, elderberry, maitake, turkey tail, shiitake, cleavers, mahonia, propolis, calendula, olive leaf, oregano, thyme, elecampane, sage, pau d'arco*

RECIPES *Bone broth (page 76); Mushroom tonic soup (page 77); Vegan mushroom broth (page 78); Immune tincture (see right); Elderberry pastilles (see opposite); Elderberry liqueur (page 82); Fire cider (page 82)*

Immune tincture

This tincture contains antiviral and immune-boosting elderberry, antimicrobial and immune-boosting echinacea, immune-modulating reishi and lymphatic-cleansing cleavers. It can be used for fighting bacterial and viral infections, or daily during cold and flu season as a preventative. All these tinctures can be found at good herbal suppliers.

50ml (2 fl oz) echinacea tincture
50ml (2 fl oz) reishi tincture
50ml (2 fl oz) elderberry tincture
50ml (2 fl oz) cleavers tincture

Measure out the tinctures and pour into a 200ml dark glass bottle. Label and date the bottle.

TO USE For day-to-day use during cold and flu season, take 5ml (1 teaspoon) of tincture in a little water 1–2 times a day. Where there is a current infection, this tincture can be taken as 5ml (1 teaspoon) in a little water every 4 hours for up to 3 days.

SHELF LIFE 1–2 years in a cool, dark place.

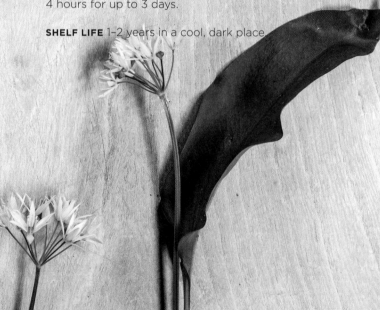

VIRAL INFECTIONS

Acute viral infections, including colds and flu, need to be fought herbally from two sides: by enhancing the action of the immune system and by taking antiviral herbs. Follow the dietary instructions for bacterial infections (opposite), and take antiviral and immune-boosting herbs in teas, syrups and tinctures. Chronic viral infections should always be treated by medical professionals.

INTERNAL HERBS *Elderberry, elderflower, echinacea, thyme, St John's wort, propolis, lemon balm, eucalyptus*

RECIPES *Bone broth (page 76); Mushroom tonic soup (page 77); Vegan mushroom broth (page 78); Immune tincture (see opposite); Fire cider (page 82); Elderberry pastilles (see right); Elderberry liqueur (page 82); Elderberry syrup (page 111)*

Elderberry pastilles

These pastilles can be used for coughs, colds, sore throats and as a general immune booster during cold and flu season.

2 tablespoons dried elderberries
1 tablespoon dried yarrow flowers
1 tablespoon dried thyme
1 teaspoon cinnamon powder
1 tablespoon marshmallow root or slippery elm powder
1–2 tablespoons honey or glycerine
3 tablespoons warm water or herbal infusion of your choice

Place all the dry ingredients in a high-powered food processor or use a pestle and mortar and blend or crush until you have a fine powder. Transfer the powder to a bowl.

Pour over the honey or glycerine and the warm water or herbal infusion, and mix well to form a paste.

ELDERBERRY

Elderberries act in a similar way to echinacea, boosting the immune system and helping to prevent viral replication in the cold and flu viruses. Unlike echinacea, it is a common wild plant, and provides abundant quantities of flowers and berries that can be dried for all year round use. Don't be tempted to eat the berries fresh though, as they can cause vomiting. However, once dried, tinctured or cooked, they are fine to use.

Elderberry liqueur

This delicious spiced elderberry liqueur contains plenty of antimicrobial and immune-boosting herbs. Take it at the first sign of cold or flu, or as a preventative if you are in an environment where infection is doing the rounds. For an alcohol-free alternative, make an elderberry syrup with elderberries and the same spices by following the instructions on page 111.

50g (1¾ oz) brown sugar
300g (10½ oz) elderberries, lightly crushed
grated zest of 1 orange
5cm (2in) piece of fresh ginger root, sliced thinly
10 cardamom pods, crushed
10 cloves, crushed
2 cinnamon sticks
port
brandy or vodka

Place the berries, fruit and spices in a large wide-mouth jar and cover with port until about one-quarter of the way up. Fill the rest of the jar with brandy or vodka and leave to infuse for 2–4 weeks.

Strain off the liquid, squeezing out and discarding the solids, then transfer the liquid to a labelled and dated dark glass bottle.

TIP This can also be made with dried berries which will need to fill the jar to a third of the way.

TO USE Take 5–10ml (1–2 teaspoons) in a little water, or with hot water, 2–3 times a day.

SHELF LIFE Due to the high alcohol content, this will keep for at least 2 years.

Fire cider

The stimulating, yet simple store-cupboard ingredients in this recipe make a warming remedy that packs a punch. It is a popular traditional remedy for a range of health benefits from improving circulation to stimulating digestion. It is also a handy for coughs and sore throats, but it is a fiery one, so it's not for the faint-hearted!

1 small onion, sliced or diced
a few sprigs of rosemary
a few sprigs of thyme
a few sprigs of sage
5 chillies
1 teaspoon cayenne/chilli pepper
5cm (2in) piece of fresh turmeric, finely sliced
10cm (4in) piece of fresh ginger root, finely sliced
5–10cm (2–4in) piece of friesh horseradish root, finely sliced
2 teaspoons black peppercorns, crushed
1 whole head of garlic, peeled and crushed
1 unwaxed lemon, sliced
1 litre (1¾ pint) raw apple cider vinegar

Layer all of the ingredients in a wide-mouth large jar (large enough to fit the ingredients and 1 litre vinegar). Pour over the apple cider vinegar. Leave to infuse for 2–4 weeks, then strain. Bottle the liquid, label and date.

NOTE this recipe will be best once left to infuse for a few weeks but if needed sooner, it can be used after a few hours of preparing – simply take a teaspoon or two as needed from the jar and leave the rest to infuse for the full 2–4 week period.

TO USE Take 2 teaspoons in a little hot or cold water. For sore throats, mix 1 teaspoon of fire cider with 1 teaspoon of honey in 4 teaspoons water, gargle and swallow

SHELF LIFE Up to one year in a cool dry place.

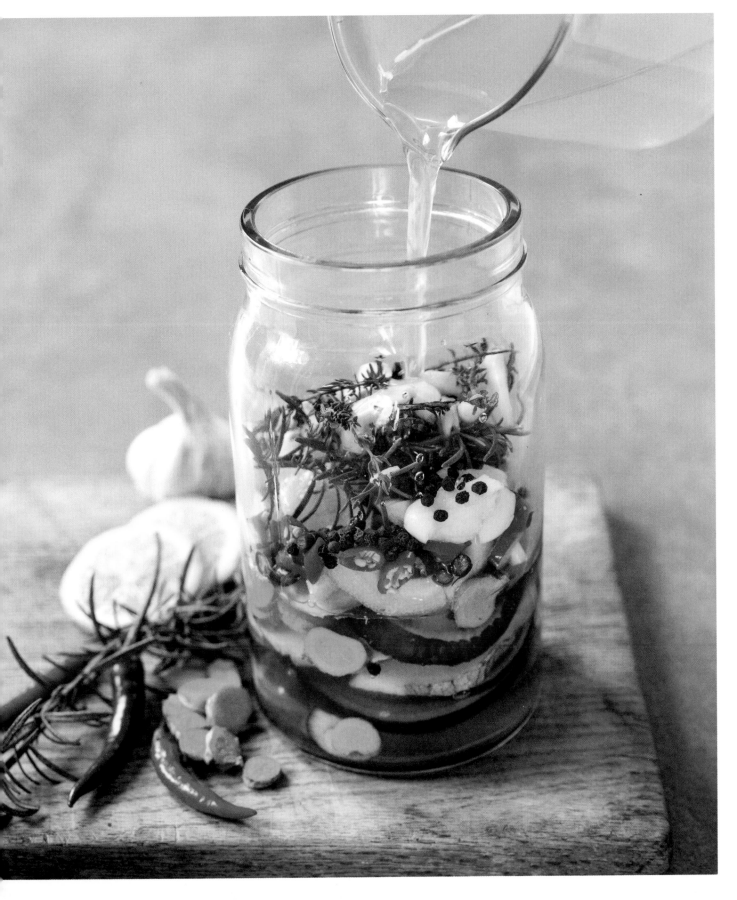

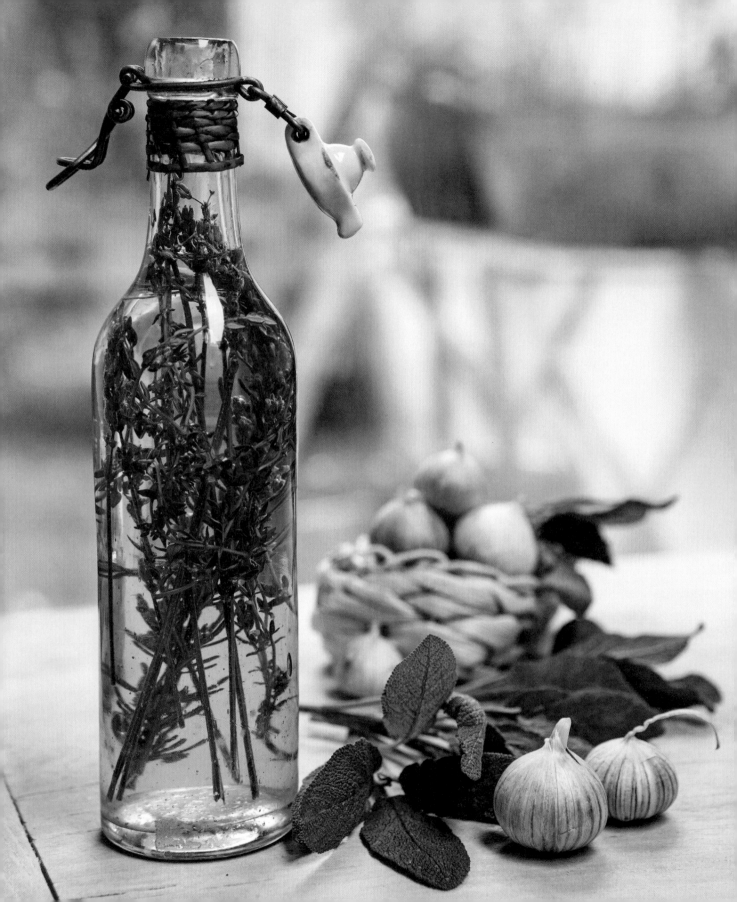

FUNGAL INFECTIONS

We all have a delicate ecosystem of naturally occurring fungi that live throughout our bodies. Fungal infections usually occur when the immune system is not working to its full capacity, allowing either our native fungi to become overgrown or an invading foreign fungus to colonise. Fungi thrive in warm, damp environments such as between the toes and in folds of skin, leading to infections such as athlete's foot and thrush. Try to wear loose-fitting clothing around the site of infection to allow for adequate air flow. Treat the immune system as a whole with internal elderberry and echinacea, along with topical antifungal herbs.

INTERNAL HERBS *Oregano, thyme, eucalyptus, calendula, echinacea, elderberry, sage, garlic, pau d'arco*

EXTERNAL HERBS *Myrrh, oregano, thyme, eucalyptus, calendula, echinacea, tea tree, sage, garlic, pau d'arco, lavender*

RECIPES *Antimicrobial gel (page 37); Immune tincture (page 80); Four thieves vinegar (see right); Antifungal powder (page 146)*

Four thieves vinegar

Legend has it that this recipe was exchanged for release from arrest by some audacious and seemingly immune looters during a plague outbreak. It has remained a popular and powerful remedy used by herbalists today – but for fungal infections such as ringworm, athlete's foot and fungal toenail rather than the black death. You can use whole stalks of herbs, if desired.

2 tablespoons fresh or dried lavender
2 tablespoons fresh or dried rosemary
2 tablespoons fresh or dried sage
2 tablespoons fresh or dried thyme
2 tablespoons fresh or dried oregano
15 cloves
2 garlic cloves, peeled and quartered
Around 500ml (18 flo oz) vinegar (a low-scent type, such as white wine or raw apple cider)

Bash or chop all the herbs. Place them in a 500ml (18 fl oz) jar and cover with vinegar. Leave to infuse for a month in a cool, dark place, shaking occasionally. Strain into a clean bottle, label and date.

TO USE Dilute the vinegar with water or a herbal infusion to a ratio of 50:50. Soak a cotton pad with the mixture and regularly wipe the affected area. Avoid the genital and eye areas. Alternatively, add 240ml (9 fl oz) of infused vinegar to 2 litres (3½ pints) of hot water and use as a foot bath. Dilute 10ml (2 teaspoons) vinegar to 20ml (4 teaspoons) water and use as a gargle for sore throats.

SHELF LIFE Up to 1 year in a cool, dark place. Discard if mouldy.

CONJUNCTIVITIS

Swelling and inflammation of the juctiva – the thin transparent layer that covers the white of the eye – causes what is commonly known as 'pink eye' or conjunctivitis. It can produce a sticky pus that gets trapped in the eyelashes, making it hard to open the eyes, especially after a period of sleep. Conjunctivitis can be contagious so ensure scrupulous hygiene to prevent it spreading to your other eye or to other people. Chamomile tea bags, brewed in boiling water and allowed to cool then placed over closed eyes, can be used as a quick anti-inflammatory eye compress.

INTERNAL HERBS *Cleavers, echinacea, elderberry, elderflower, eyebright*

RECIPES *Bone broth (page 76); Mushroom tonic soup (page 77); Vegan mushroom broth (page 78); Immune tincture (page 80); Elderberry pastilles (page 81); Elderberry liqueur (page 82); Itchy-eye cooler cubes (page 118)*

SHINGLES

Also known as herpes zoster, shingles is a painful infection of a nerve and the surrounding skin caused by the varicella-zoster virus, the same virus that causes chickenpox. The main symptom of shingles is acute pain, followed by a rash of itchy blisters, which can continue to form for up to 2 weeks. While blisters are continuing to develop, it is best to avoid oily, heating applications, instead keep the affected area clean and dry by lightly dabbing or spraying with diluted St John's wort tincture (5:1 ratio of water to tincture). The Lemon balm and St John's wort infused oil recipe opposite is perfect during the healing stage to prevent scarring. Wear loose-fitting clothes that do not irritate the rash.

Shingles is highly contagious, so stay home and maintain scrupulous hygiene, washing bedding and towels frequently and washing hands after cleaning or touching blisters. Avoid susceptible groups of people, including the elderly, pregnant women, babies and those with a weakened immune system.

INTERNAL HERBS *St John's wort, lemon balm, echinacea, thyme, elderberry*

EXTERNAL HERBS *St John's wort, lemon balm, calendula, lavender, thyme*

RECIPES *Bone broth (page 76); Mushroom tonic soup (page 77); Vegan mushroom broth (page 78); Immune tincture (page 80); Elderberry pastilles (page 81); Elderberry liqueur (page 82); Lemon balm & St John's wort infused oil (see opposite)*

Lemon balm &
St John's wort infused oil

The shingles rash may leave minor scarring: apply this oil after blisters have stopped forming to keep the skin moisturised and to aid healing. This recipe uses fresh St John's wort flowers; if fresh flowers are unavailable, buy a good-quality infused oil from your local herbal or health food shop or herbalist. The very last option is to infuse dried St John's wort herb in place of the fresh – however, it really is best fresh for this purpose!

1–2 handfuls of fresh lemon balm leaves
1–2 handfuls of fresh St John's wort flowering tops (collect unopened flower buds, flowers and the top few leaves)
olive oil
cold-pressed rosehip oil
thyme essential oil
lavender essential oil

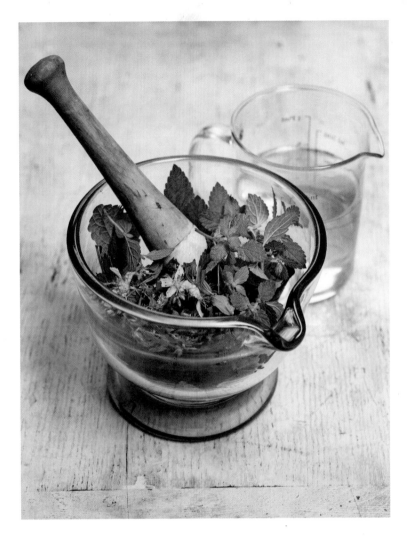

Pick your fresh herbs, lay them out on a tea towel and leave to wilt overnight out of direct sunlight or heat – this helps to remove some of the water but keeps the important essential oils which help to preserve the finished product.

Once wilted, chop the herbs finely. If using dried St John's wort, crush it slightly using a pestle and mortar.

Place all the herbs in a jar and cover with olive oil, making sure all the plant material is submerged.

If you have time, infuse the oil using the sun method (page 23), or for a quicker result, heat the oil gently in a bain-marie (page 24).

Strain off the oil through a muslin-lined sieve, discarding the plant material. Do not squeeze the muslin, instead let it drip through (squeezing will cause water from the plant material to enter the oil, which will give your oil a shorter shelf life).

Pour your resulting oil into a measuring jug. For every 10ml (2 teaspoons) of oil, add 1ml (about 20 drops) of cold-pressed rosehip oil, 1 drop of thyme essential oil and 1 drop of lavender essential oil. Bottle, label and date.

TO USE Apply 1–3 times a day to affected areas as they heal.

SHELF LIFE Store in the fridge for up to 6 months. Discard if it smells rancid.

MOOD & EMOTIONS
ANXIETY

Anxiety is a feeling of unease, worry or fear. Most people will experience some form of anxiety in their lives; like stress, it is a normal part of our physiology for survival. But it can become chronic (lasting over a long period) or extreme (causing intense feelings of anxiety that are short-lived, known as panic or anxiety attacks). It can even cause physical symptoms like mild heart palpitations, rapid breathing, sweating and muscle tension. Taking time to practise meditation and mindfulness can help. Also, take time for self-care by brewing a cup of herbal tea from a mixture of the herbs below.

INTERNAL HERBS *Chamomile, liquorice, linden flower, motherwort, hawthorn, ginseng, rose petals, skullcap, St John's wort, vervain, oatstraw, ashwagandha*

RECIPES *Anti-anxiety spray (see right); Rescue drops (see opposite)*

Anti-anxiety spray

It is not always possible to sit back, pop the kettle on and make a cup of soothing herbal tea. This aromatic spray can be kept in your bag or on your desk at work and used as needed. The olfactory nerve (responsible for our sense of smell) is linked directly to the limbic system and amygdala, the parts of the brain that control our stress response, mood, emotions and memory. Smelling some essential oils can also help to lessen rapid heart rate and other symptoms of anxiety.

80ml (2½ fl oz) distilled rose water or distilled water
10 drops lavender essential oil
10 drops geranium essential oil
10 drops mandarin essential oil
5ml (1 teaspoon) glycerine (optional)
20ml (4 teaspoons) vodka

Mix all the ingredients together in a spray bottle. Shake well before each use. Label and date.

TO USE Simply spritz a few times into the air in front of you, and step into the mist as you take a deep breath in.

SHELF LIFE Up to 3 months.

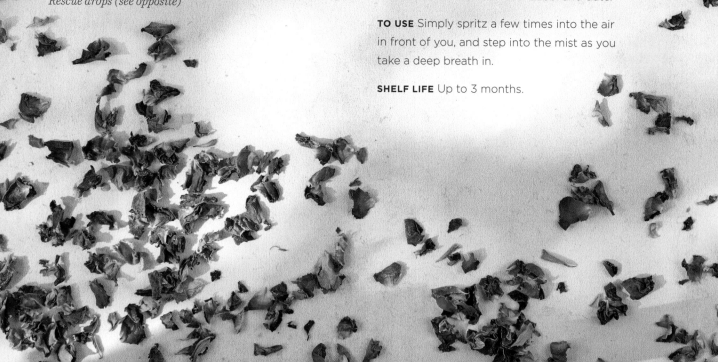

STRESS

Stress is a normal physiological reaction to our external environment. In evolutionary terms, the hormones released during stressful moments would have given us an extra push of adrenaline when trying to fight off a predator or hunt down food. However, when stress becomes long term, especially in our more sedentary, modern-day lives, it can cause havoc within the body. Taking time for self-care is extremely important. Eat properly to nourish the nervous system, exercise outside, practise yoga or meditation, and take some time for yourself. Use the Relaxing massage bars on page 93, and brew a cup of skullcap, oatstraw and chamomile tea, or a mixture of any of the herbs listed below.

INTERNAL HERBS *Chamomile, liquorice, motherwort, oatstraw, ginseng, rose petals, schisandra, skullcap, St John's wort, vervain, oatstraw, ashwagandha*

RECIPES *Anti-anxiety spray (opposite); Rescue drops (see right); Breakfast bites (page 90); Relaxing massage bars (page 93)*

Rescue drops

These drops can be used daily to support the body in times of stress, and as a stress 'rescue' for intense moments. These tinctures can be made or bought from a good herbal supplier.

50ml (2 fl oz) liquorice tincture

50ml (2 fl oz) ginseng tincture

50ml (2 fl oz) hawthorn tincture

50ml (2 fl oz) skullcap tincture

Mix the tinctures together in a 200ml (⅓ pint) dark glass bottle. Pour a little into a small bottle with a pipette and keep in your bag for when you need a moment of calm.

TO USE Take 5ml (1 teaspoon) each morning and evening. Take another 1ml (about 20 drops) for emergency moments up to 5 times a day.

SHELF LIFE Up to 2 years in a cool, dark place.

ADAPTOGENIC STRESS HERBS

These are herbs for resilience. They lift the mood and support the adrenals, improve energy levels and our body's ability to cope with stresses, and reduce 'brain fog'.

INTERNAL HERBS *Schisandra, ginseng, ashwagandha, liquorice, astragalus, cordyceps, tulsi, reishi.*

LOW ENERGY

It may seem counter-productive, but physical exercise is possibly the best way to improve low energy, especially exercise taken outside. Ensuring you eat a good variety of whole foods and are receiving all recommended protein, calories, vitamins and minerals for you is also vital. Tonic herbal infusions (page 12) can add additional nutrients to the diet. When energy levels drop, herbalists reach for a group of herbs called adaptogens (see box on page 89).

INTERNAL HERBS *Passionflower, schisandra, ginseng, ashwagandha, liquorice*

RECIPES *Fire cider (page 82); Rescue drops (page 89); Breakfast bites (see right); Focus tincture (opposite)*

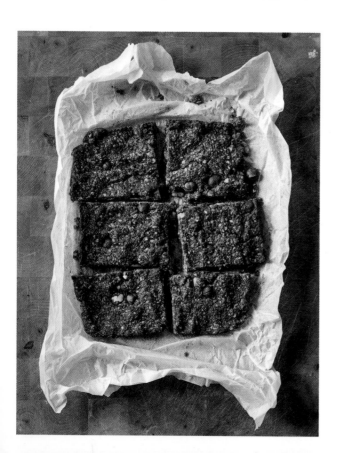

Breakfast bites

When we are stressed out or chronically tired it can be hard to muster the energy to feed ourselves properly. Start the day the right way with these herb-packed bites. They can be made in bulk and frozen, then thawed for a quick mid-morning snack or eaten with fruit as a balanced breakfast. These bites contain nutrient-dense foods, high in B vitamins, trace minerals and 'good' fats, along with adaptogenic herbal powders to support a healthy functioning nervous system.

70g (2½ oz) Brazil nuts
50g (1¾ oz) hazelnuts or almonds
1 tablespoon schisandra berries
175g (6oz) pitted dates
70g (2½ oz) rolled oats
40g (1½ oz) chopped dried fruit
1 tablespoon ashwagandha powder
30g (1oz) poppy seeds
20g (¾ oz) coconut oil
150ml (¼ pint) unsweetened apple juice or water

Preheat the oven to 180°C (350°F).

Blend the nuts (reserving a few whole), schisandra berries and dates in a high-powered blender. Scoop the paste out into a bowl and combine with the remaining ingredient, including the whole nuts. Spread the mixture evenly on a parchment-lined baking tray to about 1.5cm (⅝ in) thick and bake for 20–25 minutes. Leave to cool and then cut into 2.5–5cm (1–2 in) squares. Alternatively, use a dehydrator for 'raw' bites.

TO USE Eat 1–2 pieces a day.

SHELF LIFE Up to 2 weeks in the fridge, or 6 months in the freezer, in an airtight container.

BRAIN FOG/POOR MEMORY & CONCENTRATION

Brain fog can be experienced as forgetfulness, detachment and an inability to concentrate, and can occur during times of stress, hormonal disruption and exhaustion. There are herbs that have been used traditionally to help increase focus, concentration, lessen stress and improve blood flow to the brain.

If brain fog comes on suddenly or is severe, be sure to see a medical practitioner as it could be a sign of something more serious.

INTERNAL HERBS *Rosemary, lemon balm, schisandra, sage, gotu kola, ashwagandha, ginseng, basil, tulsi, gingko*

RECIPES *Fire cider (page 82); Rescue drops (page 89); Breakfast bites (opposite); Focus tincture (below)*

Focus tincture

Poor concentration can be frustrating when life calls for you to be on the ball. This focus tincture contains herbs that have been used for centuries to lessen stress, increase focus and improve memory and blood flow to the brain. It comes in very handy when you are not feeling at the top of your game mentally. Take it before meetings, presentations and when studying, or just when you're feeling generally brain-foggy. All these tinctures can be made at home or bought from a good herbal supplier.

20ml (4 teaspoons) schisandra tincture
20ml (4 teaspoons) gotu kola tincture
20ml (4 teaspoons) lemon balm tincture
20ml (4 teaspoons) rosemary tincture
20ml (4 teaspoons) ginseng tincture

Mix all the tinctures together in a dark glass bottle, label and date.

TO USE Shake before use. Take 5ml (1 teaspoon) of this tincture up to 3 times a day in a little water or juice.

SHELF LIFE Up to 2 years in a cool, dark place.

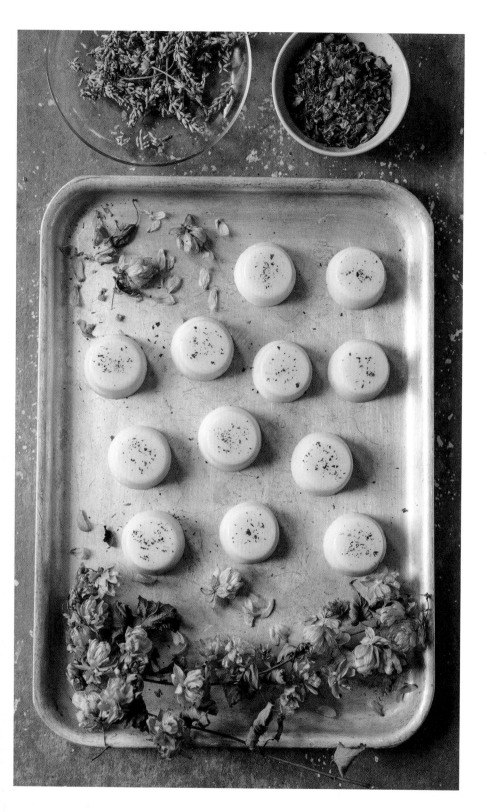

INSOMNIA

Most people suffer from a lack of sleep every now and then, but for some it is a constant battle. 'Sleep hygiene' is a popular management tool to help you psychologically prepare for sleep; this includes keeping your bed only for sleep – no TV, laptop or phone browsing – and is well worth researching as a technique. Traditional herbal recipes will not only help ease you into sleep but will also aid sleep quality and help you awake refreshed. The most famous of these is the simple European remedy of making a deep-decoction (page 13) of linden flower to drink or add to a bath.

INTERNAL HERBS *Valerian, linden flower, chamomile, oatstraw, St John's wort, lavender, passionflower, lemon balm, ashwagandha, wild lettuce*

ESSENTIAL OILS *Frankincense, lavender, ylang-ylang, lemon, rose, jasmine, mandarin, vanilla, chamomile*

Relaxing massage bars

These sweet-smelling bars have a lovely creamy consistency, perfect for massaging tense muscles before bed and giving yourself some well-deserved care. Massaging the feet well before sleep is an old and effective method to help those who find it hard to drift off. It is thought that it helps to bring blood flow down to the feet away from the head.

1 tablespoon dried or fresh rose petals

1 tablespoon dried or fresh hop flowers

1 tablespoon cardamom pods, lightly crushed

50g (1¾ oz) cocoa butter

50g (1¾ oz) shea butter

10 drops mandarin essential oil

10 drops ylang-ylang essential oil

Place the flowers, cardamom, cocoa butter and shea butter in a bain-marie (page 24) and infuse over a low heat for 2–3 hours, keeping an eye on the pan.

Take the mixture off the heat. Allow to cool slightly for 5 minutes, then strain the liquid (discard the solids), add the essential oils and pour into a soft silicone mould to set. Once cool and firm, store in an airtight container.

TO USE Massage over the body once or twice a day, concentrating on any areas of tension and stress.

SHELF LIFE Up to 1 year in an airtight container in a cool, dark place.

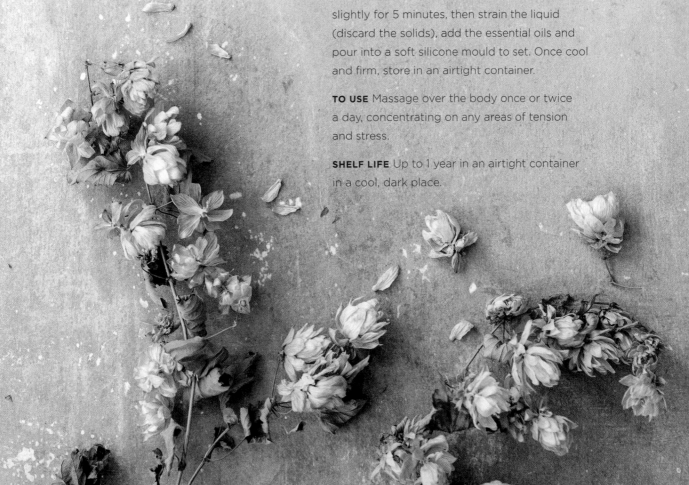

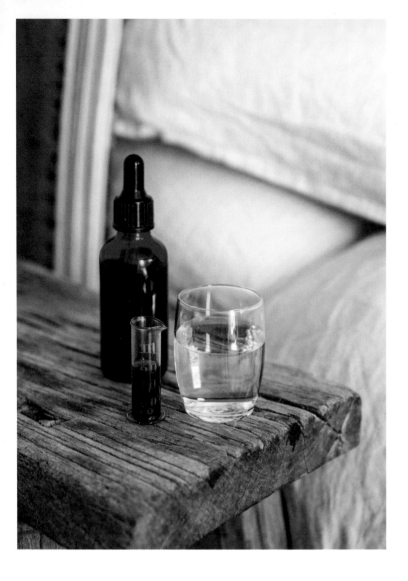

Night-time tincture

This tincture contains soothing sedative herbs that help both the body and mind drift off into a gentle slumber. It can be taken before bed, or if you are someone who wakes halfway through the night, it can be kept by the bedside table and taken to help you get back to sleep. All these tinctures can be made or bought from good herbal suppliers.

25ml (1 fl oz) wild lettuce tincture
25ml (1 fl oz) skullcap tincture
25ml (1 fl oz) linden flower tincture
25ml (1 fl oz) passionflower tincture

Mix all of the tinctures in a dark glass dropper bottle, label and date.

TO USE Take 5ml (1 teaspoon) of tincture in a little water before bed. Take another 5ml (1 teaspoon) if you wake up in the night.

SHELF LIFE Up to 2 years in a cool, dark place.

Scented sleep spray

You can use in an oil diffuser in your bedroom or in a handy spray bottle for your pillow and to spray around your room before bed.

40 drops of a mix of the following essential oils:
   lavender, frankincense, chamomile
20ml (4 teaspoons) alcohol (e.g. vodka)
80ml (2½ fl oz) filtered water

Add the essential oil to the alcohol in a 100ml (3½ fl oz) spray bottle, mix well, then top up with filtered water.

TO USE Spray around the room and step into the mist, or spray onto bedding from a distance.

SHELF LIFE Up to 6 months in a cool, dark place.

Cardamom, rose & linden cocoa

Relaxing, sleep-inducing herbs are infused with almond milk and cocoa, both of which contain the amino acid tryptophan, which encourages the production of sleep-enhancing chemicals. This evening drink should help you drift gently away.

2 cardamom pods, lightly crushed
1 teaspoon each of rose petals, linden
    flowers and ashwagandha powder
1 tablespoon cocoa powder
300ml (½ pint) almond milk
sugar, honey or fruit syrup, to taste

Place all the ingredients into a small pan. Cover and simmer gently for 10–15 minutes. Remove from the heat and strain. Allow to sit for a further 10–15 minutes until cool enough to sip. Serve immediately, ideally an hour before bedtime.

TO USE Drink 1 cup before bed.

SHELF LIFE Use immediately.

TIP The dried elements of the recipe can be gathered in bulk, whizzed in a power blender (take the seeds out of the cardamom pods) and kept in a cool, dark place. Use 2 teaspoons per mug of hot milk, as needed.

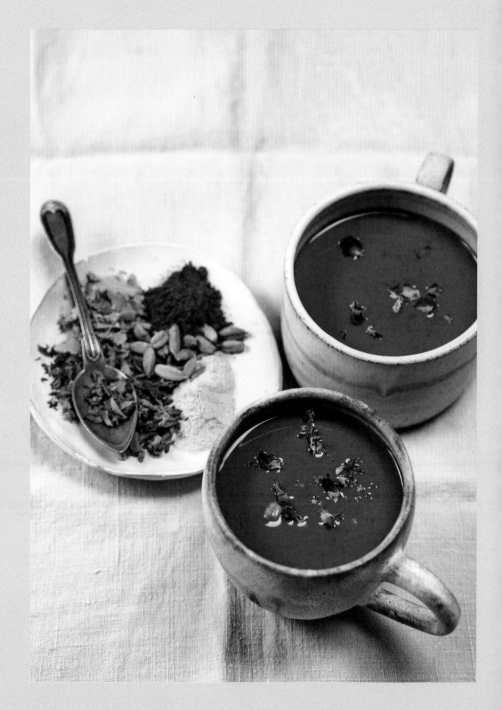

MUSCLES, BONES & JOINTS
ARTHRITIS

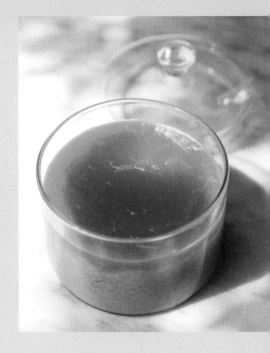

There are two main forms of arthritis: osteo and rheumatoid. Osteoarthritis is caused by wear and tear of the cartilage and bone, while rheumatoid arthritis is an autoimmune condition where the body's own immune system attacks the connective tissues around the joints. The two have different origins, and to treat the underlying cause it may be worth visiting a herbalist for a holistic approach. Both forms of arthritis share similar symptoms of pain and inflammation, so herbal home remedies aim to reduce these symptoms.

Herbs high in antioxidants and other anti-inflammatory compounds such as turmeric or rosehip can be taken daily, either in the diet, or in tincture or capsule form. Having a healthy diet is key to maintaining healthy tissues and reducing the negative symptoms of arthritis: keep deep-fried foods to a minimum and omega-3 oils high. Eat a rainbow diet high in vitamins, minerals, antioxidants and 'good' fats; these help to prevent inflammation and damage to tissues. Drink long/overnight infusions (page 12) of herbs such as nettle or cleavers, which are high in essential bone minerals such as calcium, magnesium and silica.

INTERNAL HERBS *Turmeric, cayenne, black pepper, devil's claw, red clover, nettle, horsetail, meadowsweet, willow bark, cleavers, rosehip, burdock, dandelion, celery seed, cat's claw*

EXTERNAL HERBS *Comfrey, chilli, willow bark, ginger, mustard, black pepper*

RECIPES *Nettle soup (page 54); Bone broth (page 76); Chilli & ginger joint rub (see right); Nettle and mushroom concentrate powder (page 103); Comfrey balm (page 104)*

Chilli & ginger joint rub

Cayenne pepper encourages blood flow to tissues when applied locally, which can aid in the removal of inflammation and pain. Capsaicin, a major constituent of chilli peppers, has been shown to block certain receptors in the nervous system responsible for the sensation of pain.

Use this balm on painful joints and muscles, but take care as chilli packs a punch! It will cause warming in the area it is applied to, so wash hands after use and do not get any in the eyes or genital area – it will sting!

300g (10½ oz) coconut oil
thumb-sized piece of fresh ginger root, sliced thinly
10g (¼ oz) black pepper seeds, crushed

Place the coconut oil, ginger and pepper in a bain-marie (page 24) and infuse over a low heat for 2–4 hours.
Strain the mixture while still warm using a muslin-lined sieve. Discard the solids, then pour into labelled and dated jars.

TO USE Apply a little balm to aching muscles and joints, massaging in well. Wash hands after use.

SHELF LIFE Up to 1 year.

BACK ACHE

A bad back can really affect overall wellness and make daily activities near impossible. Causes include damage to a muscle, ligament, nerve or spinal disc. Seek medical advice before treating at home if pain is extreme or chronic. The main aim of herbal treatment is to ease pain and inflammation, and herbs can be used topically and internally for this purpose. If sciatica is the cause of the pain, try an infused oil or balm made of St John's wort, as it is specific for nerve pain. Where muscles are the primary cause of pain, try a balm made from elder or comfrey infused oils.

INTERNAL HERBS *Turmeric, cayenne, St John's wort, skullcap*

EXTERNAL HERBS *Elder leaf, comfrey, lavender, cayenne, St John's wort, ginger, bay leaf, pine needle*

RECIPES *Chilli & ginger joint rub (see opposite); Ache-ease liniment (see left); Muscle-ease tincture (page 99); Comfrey balm (page 104)*

Ache-ease liniment

This liniment uses alcohol and oil infused with herbs, which when massaged over the skin of inflamed joints can help to bring blood flow to the local area and reduce inflammation.

50ml (2 fl oz) comfrey tincture
30ml (1 fl oz) bay leaf tincture
20ml (4 teaspoons) black pepper tincture
100ml (3½ fl oz) St John's wort infused oil
40 drops sweet birch or wintergreen essential oil

Mix all the ingredients together, shake well to combine, then transfer to a labelled and dated bottle. Be sure to label 'not for internal use'.

TO USE The mixture will naturally separate into oil and alcohol, so shake well before each use. Rub a small amount of the liniment over sore areas 1–3 times a day.

SHELF LIFE Up to 1 year in a cool, dark place.

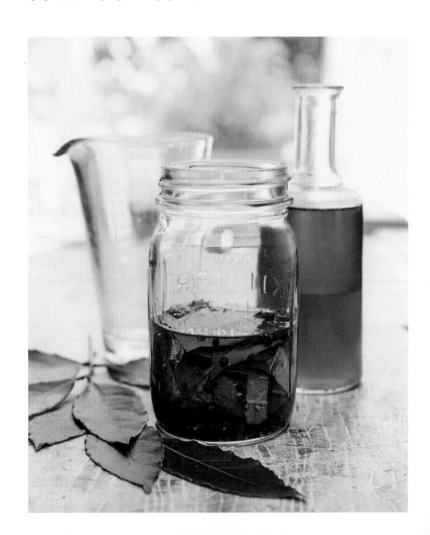

SCIATICA

Sciatica is characterised by pain from a nerve running from the lower back down the leg. Onset is usually sudden after activities such as heavy lifting, a fall or strenuous exercise. The best thing for sciatica is rest and gentle stretching along with warm herbal compresses. Sciatica should clear up on its own in 4–6 weeks with rest and treatment; if pain is severe or chronic, seek medical attention to rule out a herniated disc or other underlying causes.

INTERNAL HERBS *St John's wort, skullcap, meadowsweet, turmeric*

EXTERNAL HERBS *St John's wort, ginger, black pepper, chilli, mustard*

RECIPES *Ache-ease liniment (page 97); St John's wort compress (see below); Muscle-ease tincture (opposite); Comfrey balm (page 104)*

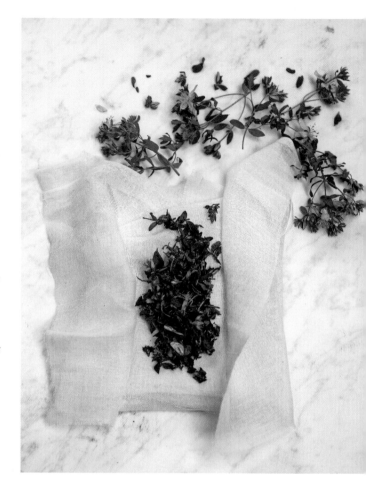

St John's wort compress

St John's wort has a long traditional use of relieving nerve pain. It has a variety of constituents, including hyperforin, which help reduce inflammation and improve tissue healing when applied topically. St John's wort tea or tincture can also be taken internally for this purpose, but it can interact with some medications and should not be used during pregnancy.

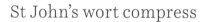

St John's wort infused oil or fresh St John's wort herb
Gauze/Muslin
Bandages
Clingfilm
Towel
Hot water bottle

COMPRESS METHOD Soak a gauze or bandage in St John's wort infused oil. Apply to the affected area then wrap with another bandage to keep in place. To prevent things getting messy, you can then apply a layer of clingfilm. Place a towel and hot water bottle over the compress and relax with it in place for at least 30 minutes.

POULTICE METHOD Take a large handful of fresh St John's wort (flowering tops), mash using a pestle and mortar and sandwich between 2 layers of muslin. Apply to the affected area, cover with clingfilm and place a hot water bottle over the compress. Leave in place for at least 30 minutes.

TO USE Apply 1-2 times a day.

SHELF LIFE Use immediately.

MUSCLE & JOINT PAIN

The most common cause of mild joint and muscle pain is from injury or overuse. Being overweight can also put excess pressure on joints, causing the wearing down of cartilage, potentially leading to arthritis and severe pain. Rest, compresses and warm healing baths with herbs can help to alleviate the pain of aching muscles and joints. Try taking tissue-healing and anti-inflammatory herbs such as turmeric and meadowsweet internally too.

INTERNAL HERBS *Cramp bark, St John's wort, rosemary, cayenne, black pepper, meadowsweet, willow bark, ginger, turmeric*

EXTERNAL HERBS *Cayenne, St John's wort, comfrey, black pepper, ginger, lavender, rosemary, pine needle*

RECIPES *Chilli & ginger joint rub (page 96); St John's wort compress (page 98); Muscle-ease tincture (see right); Herbal muscle soak (page 100); Comfrey balm (page 104)*

Muscle-ease tincture

The clue is in the name of the herb: cramp bark can help to relax tired and spasming muscles, reducing pain. It is useful for menstrual and muscular cramps.

200g (7oz) cramp bark, finely chopped or powdered
50g (1¾ oz) fresh ginger root, sliced
vodka

Make a basic tincture by placing the cramp bark and fresh ginger in a jar and covering with vodka. Leave for 2–4 weeks, then strain into a labelled and dated bottle.

TO USE Take 5ml (1 teaspoon) in a little water up to 3 times a day.

CURCUMINOIDS

Curcuminoids, one of the active anti-inflammatory constituents of turmeric, are best absorbed in the body with fats or piperine (a constituent found in black pepper), so when eating turmeric add plenty of black pepper and combine with cold-pressed seed or nut oils or nuts. And when buying a turmeric supplement, look out for brands that combine turmeric with piperine.

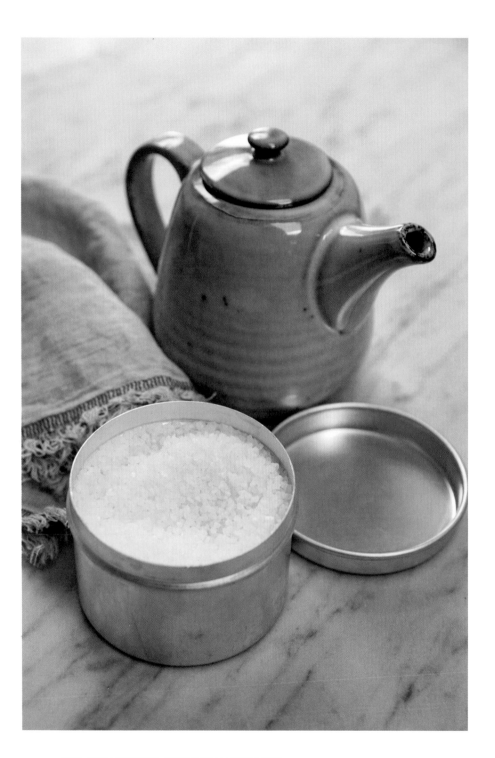

Herbal muscle soak

To alleviate tiredness and pain, try this relaxing herbal salt bath recipe using circulatory rosemary and anti-inflammatory meadowsweet.

2 heaped tablespoons dried or fresh lavender flowers
2 heaped tablespoons dried or fresh rosemary leaves
2 heaped tablespoons dried or fresh pine needles
2 heaped tablespoons meadowsweet flowers
1.5 litres (2½ pints) boiling water
300–600g (10½ oz–1lb 5oz) magnesium or Epsom salts

Make a strong infusion from the herbs by placing them in a large teapot or saucepan with the water, and allow to sit until tepid.

Strain the infusion, discarding the solids and retaining the liquid.

Pour the salts and strained herbal infusion into a bath while the water is running.

TO USE Relax in the bath for 30–45 minutes at least once a week.

SPRAINS & STRAINS

Sprains and strains are common injuries that affect muscles and ligaments. Sprains occur when ligaments around joints are stretched, twisted or torn, causing pain, swelling and bruising. For minor sprains, keep the affected joint moving with gentle stretching (only when not too painful) to prevent things ceasing up. Sprains can take a long time to heal, so long-term stretching, rest and treatment are necessary.

RICE – rest, ice, compression and elevation – are the best things for a sprain or strain, along with healing herbal poultices. Massage the affected area with an infused oil of St John's wort and comfrey with a few drops of lavender or sweet birch essential oils.

INTERNAL HERBS *St John's wort, oatstraw, nettle, calendula, turmeric, cramp bark*

EXTERNAL HERBS *Arnica, comfrey, St John's wort, black pepper, ginger, cayenne, daisy, elder leaf, sage*

RECIPES *Chilli & ginger joint rub (page 96); Ache-ease liniment (page 97); St John's wort compress (page 98); Sage vinegar poultice (see right); Comfrey balm (page 104)*

Sage vinegar poultice

This traditional recipe uses vinegar, which is said to bring bruises to the surface, and sage, which is a circulatory stimulant. It can also be used for muscle aches and pains. Try a chilled version for headaches by soaking a flannel in the refrigerated mixture and placing over the forehead.

a handful of fresh sage leaves
apple cider vinegar

Crush the sage leaves lightly using a pestle and mortar. Place in a small pan and cover with vinegar. Simmer very gently over a low heat for 5 minutes. Allow to cool to a bearable heat, then place the strained sage leaves in between two layers of muslin or bandage to create a poultice.

TO USE Apply to the affected area, at a hot but not scalding temperature. Cover with towels and leave in place for 1 hour while you relax.

SHELF LIFE Use immediately.

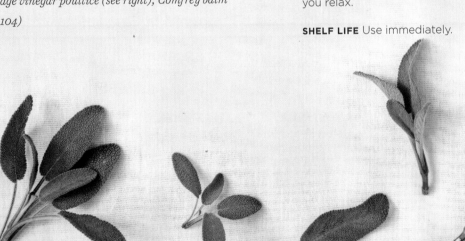

MUSCLE CRAMP

GOUT

Cramping muscles usually occur after intense exertion, or during the night in the legs and feet. Causes include lack of oxygen to the muscles, lactic acid build-up, or lack of electrolytes, including sodium, calcium, magnesium and potassium. Stretching after exercise can significantly reduce cramping, as can staying well hydrated with electrolyte-rich drinks. Try massaging tense muscles with an infused oil or balm containing warming herbs.

INTERNAL HERBS *Cramp bark, skullcap, yarrow*

EXTERNAL HERBS *Lavender, elder leaf, chilli, ginger, mustard, St John's wort, black pepper*

RECIPES *Circulation tonic tea (page 58); Horse chestnut & yarrow balm (page 61); Oral rehydration salts (page 71); Chilli & ginger joint rub (page 96); Ache-ease liniment (page 97); Muscle-ease tincture (page 99); Herbal muscle soak (page 100)*

Gout is a form of inflammatory arthritis characterised by pain caused by the build-up of uric acid crystals that form around the joints, most commonly the big toes. It is often short-lived, with attacks lasting just a week or so. Obesity, weight gain and excess alcohol consumption can all cause and worsen symptoms of gout. Avoid food high in purines, which can cause a build-up of uric acid in the body: these include red meat, liver and kidneys. Stopping smoking and taking regular exercise can also help to reduce attacks of gout. Though the area may be too painful to touch, 2–5 drops of lavender or peppermint essential oils to 1 teaspoon of sunflower or olive oil can be massaged lightly around the area. Alternatively, add this mixture of oils to a foot bath.

INTERNAL HERBS *Celery seed, dandelion leaves, meadowsweet, willow bark, cleavers*

OSTEOPOROSIS

The term 'osteoporosis' translates quite literally as 'porous bones' and refers to loss of bone tissue, measured as 'bone density'. It leads to fragile bones that are more likely to fracture, and affects women more commonly than men. It occurs particularly after the menopause, when hormone levels associated with bone maintenance reduce. It is important to eat foods high in minerals essential for bone health such as calcium, zinc, magnesium, boron, as well as vitamins C, D and K. Examples include dandelion leaves, chicory, spinach and watercress. Try long/overnight infusions (page 12) of mineral-rich herbs such as nettle, horsetail and red clover. Bitter herbs can be taken before meals to help increase vital mineral absorption.

INTERNAL HERBS *Red clover, nettle, horsetail, alfalfa, oatstraw, dandelion leaf, calendula, horsetail, cleavers, chickweed*

RECIPES *Bitter drops (page 66); Bone broth (page 76); Nettle & mushroom concentrate powder (see left)*

Nettle & mushroom concentrate powder

This powder uses dehydrated nettles, rich in the minerals that the bones need for repair and strength. Mushrooms can be laid out, gill side-up, for a few hours in the sun to increase their vitamin D content, an essential vitamin for bone health, which increases the absorption of calcium and magnesium. This recipe makes a really tasty condiment that doubles as a mineral booster.

1 colander full of freshly dried nettles
400g (14oz) white or chesnut mushrooms
10g (¼ oz) garlic powder
10g (¼ oz) sea or rock salt

Dry the mushrooms by slicing finely and placing in a low oven on a baking sheet or in a dehydrator. Once dry, place all the ingredients in a high-powered blender and whizz up until you get a fine powder.

TO USE Sprinkle 1–2 teaspoons into your food each day.

SHELF LIFE Up to 6 months in an airtight container stored in a cool, dark place.

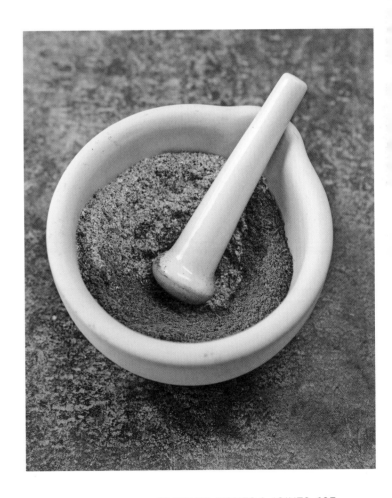

FRACTURES

Fractures and broken bones must be X-rayed and treated by a medical professional, but their healing can be aided with the use of vulnerary, tissue-healing plants. Drink long infusions (page 12) of mineral-rich plants such as nettle, red clover and horsetail.

INTERNAL HERBS *Nettle, horsetail, red clover, dandelion leaf, oatstraw, St John's wort, calendula*

EXTERNAL HERBS *Comfrey, St John's wort, elder leaf, horsetail*

Comfrey balm

Comfrey is also known as 'knitbone' and contains allantoin, which aids in the healing of tissues and has long been used traditionally to mend broken bones.

2 handfuls of dried, crumbled comfrey leaves
140ml (¼ oz) olive oil
20g (¾ oz) beeswax
20 drops rosemary essential oil
20 drops lavender essential oil

Place the dried comfrey in a bain-marie (page 24), cover with olive oil and heat gently for around 4 hours to make an infused oil.

Strain out the plant material and discard, then add the beeswax to the oil mix in the bain-marie and stir until melted. Add the essential oils and pour into a suitable jar, label and date.

TO USE Apply the ointment to the affected area 2–3 times a day.

SHELF LIFE Keep in a cool, dark place for up to 1 year.

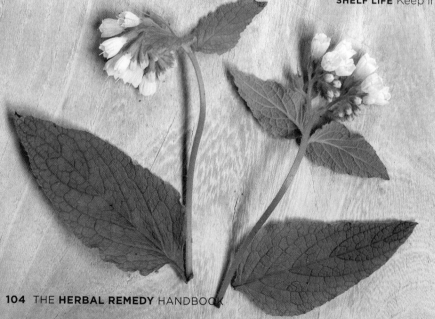

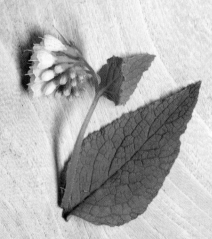

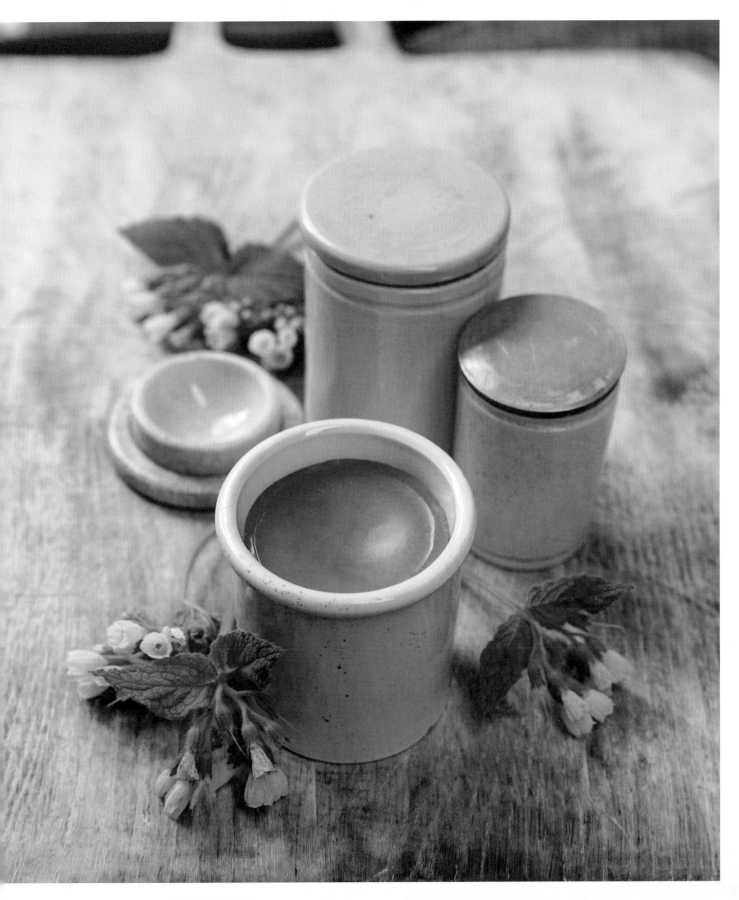

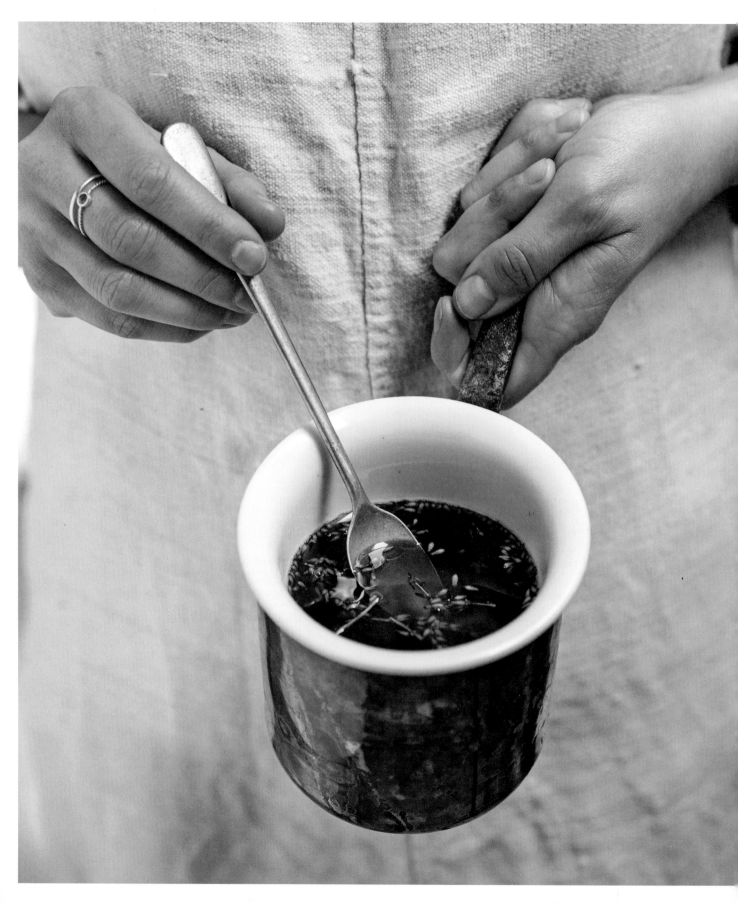

RESPIRATORY HEALTH
ASTHMA

Asthma is a breathing difficulty caused by muscle spasms in the chest and airways, which can range in severity from a mild to severe attack; emergency medical help will be required immediately in the latter. Causes of asthma can include allergies, infection, food and hereditary factors. Herbal treatment will need the guidance of a qualified professional, but traditional remedies include infusions of herbs used to support the lungs, such as thyme and elecampane.

INTERNAL HERBS *Thyme, mullein, liquorice, plantain, wild cherry bark, elecampane, sage, garlic, honeysuckle, aniseed*

RECIPES *Immune tincture (page 80); Elderberry pastilles (page 87); Decongestant chest rub (see right); Cough syrup/drops (pages 112, 115)*

Decongestant chest rub

This rub uses comfrey to help heal sore muscles that are aching due to coughing, as well as decongestant essential oils that will help relax the airways and aid breathing.

150g (5½ oz) coconut oil
1 tablespoon dried lavender flowers
1 handful of dried comfrey leaves
3 tablespoons dried thyme, chopped and crushed
4 large dried eucalyptus leaves, chopped and crushed
40–60 drops of a mix of your choice of the following essential oils: thyme, eucalyptus, tea tree, frankincense, peppermint, lavender

Heat the coconut oil gently in a bain-marie (page 24) with the lavender, comfrey, thyme and eucalyptus until the oil is well infused, aromatic and green (about 2–4 hours). Do not allow the pan to boil dry.

Remove the mixture from the heat and allow to cool for a few minutes, but not set. Using a muslin-lined sieve, strain into a jug, discarding the herbs (take care, this will be hot!). Pour the liquid into jars and allow to cool for a few more minutes.

Finally, stir in the essential oils with a cocktail stick and place the lid on to set. This will allow the essential oils to be retained in the jar rather than evaporating away with the heat. Label and date the jar.

TO USE Rub a generous amount into the chest and back, and relax.

SHELF LIFE Up to 1 year in a cool, dark place. Discard if product smells rancid or the fragrance reduces.

COLDS, FLU & CONGESTION

Mild viral infections that cause colds and flu make regular rounds during the winter. While the illness will go away on its own, traditional home remedies can help soothe symptoms and support the immune system. Elderflower and elderberries are a traditional remedy for colds and flu, and research has supported this, showing that compounds found in the plant prevent viruses from invading cells and replicating. The main herbal approach to treating colds and flu is to support the immune system (see the Immune section on page 76). The Cold & flu infusion (right) is a traditional mix of herbs helping to combat the infection. You should also increase your intake of garlic and vitamin C. A simple lemon and ginger tea can help soothe the airways and warm the body when suffering from cold and flu.

INTERNAL HERBS *Echinacea, elderberry, linden flower, garlic*

RECIPES *Steam inhalation (page 19); Immune tincture (page 80); Elderberry liqueur (page 82); Fire cider (page 82); Elderberry pastilles (page 87); Decongestant chest rub (page 107); Cold & flu infusion (see right); Chapped skin balm (see opposite); Elderberry syrup (page 111); Three herb & onion cough syrup (page 112); Cough drops (page 115); Sore throat gargle (page 119); Ginger & honey throat melts (page 120);*

Cold & flu infusion

This blend of herbs is a traditional remedy for helping colds and flu. Take it hot and head to bed for a restful and healing sleep.

20g (¾ oz) dried elderflowers
20g (¾ oz) dried elderberries
20g (¾ oz) dried yarrow
20g (¾ oz) dried peppermint leaves
few slices of fresh ginger root

Combine all the dried herbs together and store in a labelled and dated airtight container.

TO USE Place 2 teaspoons in 200ml (⅓ pint) boiling water, add a few slices of fresh ginger, if desired, cover with a lid and allow to steep for 10–15 minutes before drinking. Repeat up to 3 times a day.

SHELF LIFE Up to 1 year in a cool, dark place.

Chapped skin balm

A soft balm for that dry, chapped skin that develops around the lips and nose after a walk in the cold or after blowing your nose too often. The calendula petals encourage skin regeneration, while the shea butter and jojoba oils bring moisture to the area and create a protective barrier.

2 teaspoons dried calendula petals

2 teaspoons dried marshmallow root

20g (¾ oz) shea butter

30ml (1 fl oz) jojoba oil

2 teaspoons beeswax

½ teaspoon honey (optional)

4 drops lavender essential oil (optional)

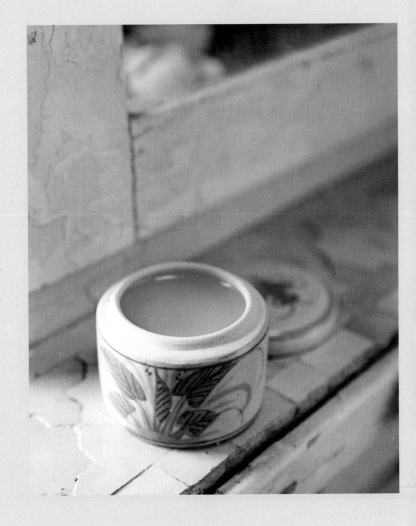

Using the bain-marie method (page 24), infuse your herbs, shea butter and oil over a gentle heat for 2–3 hours.

Remove the mixture from the heat, then strain out the petals. Return it to the bain marie and melt in the beeswax. Remove from the heat, allow to cool for a few minutes and whisk in the honey and lavender essential oil, if using. Transfer the mixture to lip balm tubs (tubs, not tubes, as this is a soft balm) or pots, then label and date.

TO USE Apply a little as needed to the nose, lips and any other dry areas of skin.

SHELF LIFE Up to 2 years in a cool, dark place.

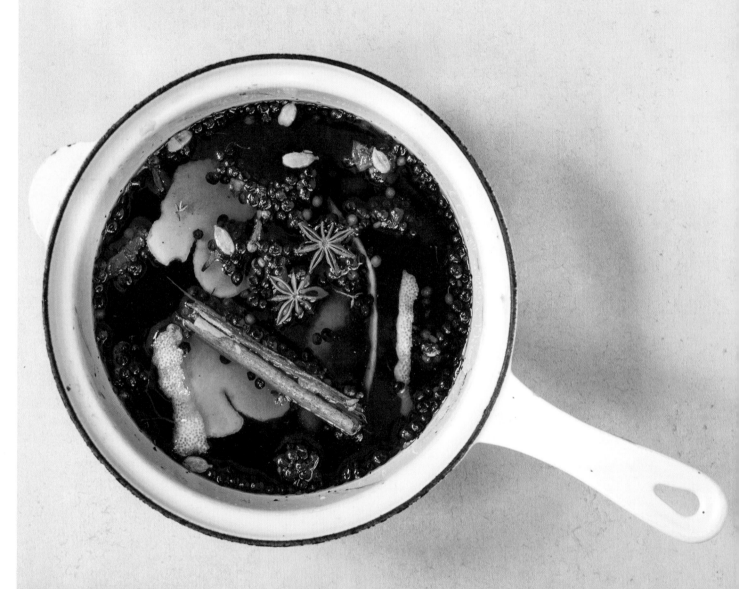

Elderberry syrup

Spiced elderberry syrup is a tasty remedy for helping to combat colds, flu, coughs and sore throats. It is also delicious used as a cordial in hot water or drizzled on ice cream.

400g (14oz) fresh or 250g (9oz) dried elderberries
1 thumb-sized piece of fresh ginger root, sliced thinly
1 cinnamon stick
2 star anise
6 cloves
6 cardamoms
6 peppercorns
zest of 1 unwaxed lemon
500ml (18 fl oz) water
approx. 500g (1lb 2oz) sugar
1 teaspoon citric acid per 500ml (18 fl oz)

Place the elderberries, spices, lemon zest and water (if using dried elderberries, add an extra 100ml (3½ fl oz) of water) in a pan. Bring to the boil and allow to simmer, uncovered, for about 20–30 minutes, until the elderberries have released their purple juices and the water has reduced by about one-third. Strain the berries through a muslin-lined sieve into a measuring jug, pressing or squeezing them to get all of the juices out.

Measure your liquid and return to the pan. For every 100ml (3½ fl oz) of liquid, add 50–100g (1¾–3½ oz) of sugar. The more sugar you add, the thicker, sweeter and more preserved your syrup will be. Bring to a gentle simmer and stir regularly until thickened and glossy. Measure the liquid, stir in the citric acid until dissolved. Pour into sterilised jars or bottles, label and date.

TO USE Take 1–2 teaspoons as necessary. Alternatively, stir 2–4 teaspoons into hot water for a soothing herbal drink.

SHELF LIFE For up to 1 year in a cool, dark place, unopened. Discard if mouldy. Once opened, keep in the fridge and use within 1 month.

Congestion and stuffiness are caused by allergies, bacterial or viral infections, inflammation and mucus production of the upper respiratory tract (throat, nose, sinus passages). Boost the immune system using echinacea and elderberry to help the body fight infection. If congestion is caused by cold and flu, see page 108 on how to treat the underlying cause. Herbal steam inhalations (page 19) using the fresh herbs and essential oils listed below are a great way to deliver decongestant, antimicrobial essential oils direct to the airways, relax the respiratory tract and bring symptomatic relief.

INTERNAL HERBS *Echinacea, elderberry, elderflower, thyme, liquorice, garlic, ground ivy, plantain, eucalyptus, sage*

EXTERNAL HERBS *(in steam inhalations) Thyme, eucalyptus, rosemary, sage*

ESSENTIAL OILS (EXTERNAL) *Thyme, eucalyptus, tea-tree, lavender (see guide on page 49)*

RECIPES *Steam inhalation (page 19); Immune tincture (page 80); Elderberry pastilles (page 81); Fire cider (page 82); Decongestant chest rub (page 107); Cold & flu infusion (page 108); Three herb & onion cough syrup (page 112)*

RESPIRATORY HEALTH **111**

COUGHS

Coughs are a natural reflex action in response to either the lungs trying to remove phlegm and mucus (wet cough), or due to inflammation and irritation (dry cough). Causes include infection, such as a cold, or an allergy, such as hay fever. Support the immune system (page 74) to help fight underlying infection, or soothe irritated membranes with moistening, cooling herbs such as marshmallow. Productive coughs that help bring up phlegm can be supported with expectorant herbs such as thyme, liquorice and elecampane, which support the mucus-removing action of the lungs. For dry (non-productive) irritated coughs that prevent restful sleep, cherry bark syrup can be taken to soothe and relax the airways.

CAUTION Whooping cough (intense periods of coughing signified by a whooping sound) and croup (cough with a barking or seal-like sound) in children can be more serious and advice should be sought from a healthcare practitioner. Bronchitis is a more chronic cough and will also need further help from a healthcare practitioner.

INTERNAL HERBS *Thyme, elecampane, mullein, liquorice, aniseed, marshmallow, garlic, elderberry, echinacea*

RECIPES *Immune tincture (page 80); Elderberry pastilles (page 81); Fire cider (page 82); Decongestant chest rub (page 107); Cold & flu infusion (page 108); Cough syrup/drops (pages 112, 115); Three herb & onion cough syrup (see right)*

Three herb & onion cough syrup

This handy store-cupboard-basics recipe can be made with just onion and sugar, if needed. The onion brings anti-infective and expectorant properties to the soothing syrup, which coats the airways. The aromatic herbs add antibacterial, expectorant and decongestant benefits and make it extra tasty, too.

1 onion, finely chopped
2 garlic cloves, finely chopped
   (optional – can be strong-tasting)
1 tablespoon finely chopped fresh thyme
1 tablespoon finely chopped fresh sage
1 tablespoon finely chopped fresh oregano
honey or sugar

Layer the onion, garlic (if using) and herbs in a jar in finger-width-sized layers alternated with equal layers of sugar. If using honey instead of sugar, simply add all the ingredients to a jar and pour the honey over to cover.

Allow to infuse until the liquid leaves the onion and a syrup mixture forms. This will happen quite quickly and the liquid 'cough syrup' can be taken as soon as this happens. However, for best results, infuse overnight or up to a week in the fridge before straining and discarding the solids using a sieve. If using honey, this may solidify in the fridge, in which case simply place the jar in a warm bowl of water before straining.

TO USE Take 1–2 teaspoons, as needed.

SHELF LIFE Use within 1 month and discard if mould forms.

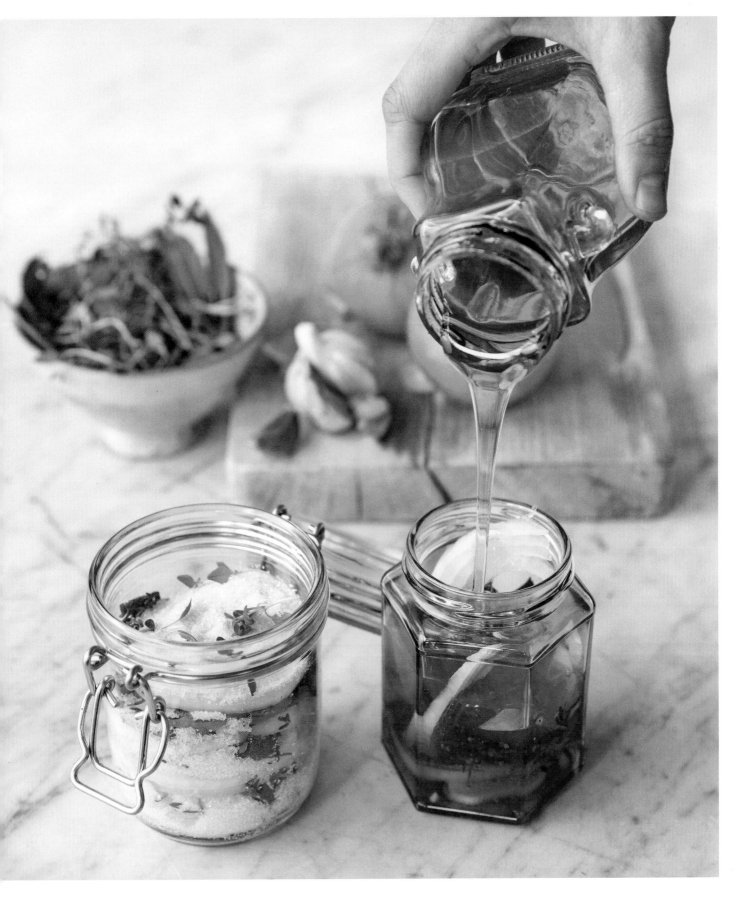

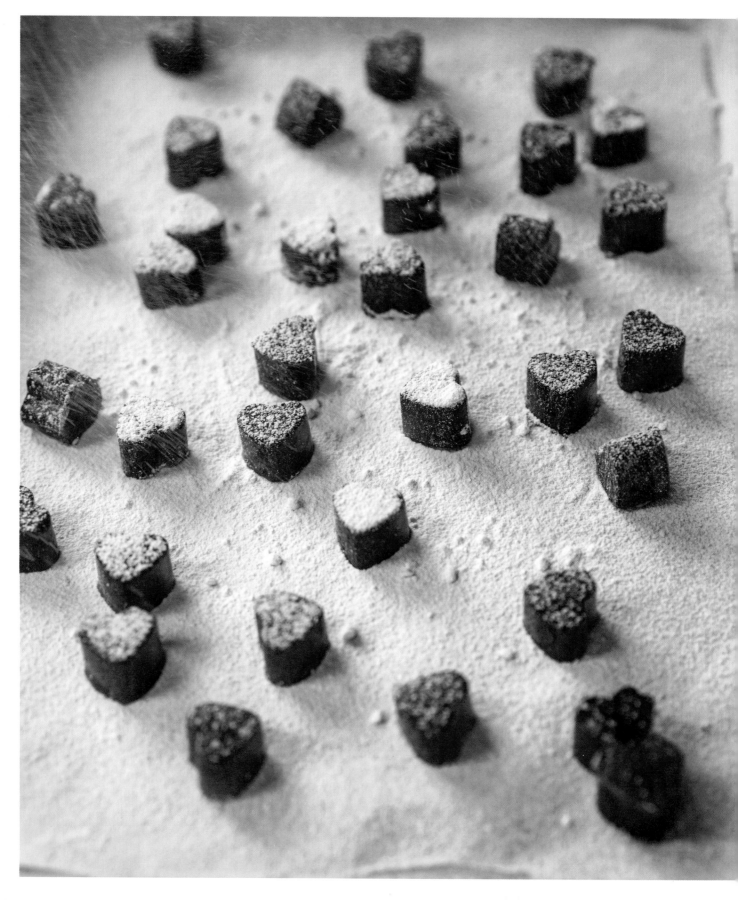

Herbal cough drops

These cough drops will take the edge off coughs, soothe achy throats and won't be hard to persuade the kids to take.

TO MAKE THE DECOCTION
50g (1¾ oz) chopped fresh ginger root

5 tablespoons aniseeds

350ml (12 fl oz) water

6–8 tablespoons chopped fresh thyme

TO MAKE THE COUGH DROPS
240ml (9 fl oz) herbal decoction (see above)

200g (7oz) granulated light brown sugar

16 tablespoons honey

STEP 1: MAKE THE DECOCTION
Place the ginger, aniseeds and water in a pan, cover with a lid and bring to a gentle simmer for 5 minutes. Remove from the heat, add the thyme, cover and allow to sit for 15 minutes. Strain, discard the spices and herbs and set aside the liquid.

STEP 2: MAKING THE DROPS
This stage uses the same method for making candy, or hard-boiled sweets. The sugar temperatures get very hot, so take care and prepare your candy moulds in advance. Use silicone moulds (not plastic!) placed on a chopping board or tray. (If you do not have this type of mould, in a baking tray, pour powdered icing sugar to a depth of 2.5cm (1in). Use a cork, a small measuring spoon or a 'sweet' shape to press little moulds into the icing. Do not push through the icing all the way to the tray.) Also have a heatproof measuring jug to hand for pouring the finished mixture.

Making candy is tricky and it really helps if you use a sugar thermometer to get the correct temperature. Place 1 cup of the decoction, sugar and honey in a large heavy-bottomed pan. Make sure the pan is large enough for the sugar to rise up when it boils.

Turn on the heat to medium-high, then stir with a wooden spoon to dissolve the sugar and honey into the liquid. Once everything has dissolved, only stir occasionally and regularly check the temperature. Make sure you stir all the way to the bottom, but avoid the sides of the pan as you do not want to mix in any crystallised sugar as it affects the finished clarity of the cough drops. Once the temperature reaches 120°C (250°F), start stirring constantly, but gently. Keep an eye on the sugar temperature because as soon as it hits 150°C (300°F), you need to immediately remove the pan from the hob using an oven mitt.

Immediately, carefully pour the hot mixture into the heatproof jug, then moving quickly, pour the liquid into the candy moulds (or the icing-sugar moulds). Allow to set overnight before removing from the moulds.

Coat in icing sugar, and store spread out in single layers separated by baking paper in an airtight container.

TO USE Suck one as needed.

SHELF LIFE Homemade candy will get softer over time, so is best used within a month.

EARACHE

HAYFEVER & ALLERGIC RHINITIS

Earache can be caused by a bacterial or viral infection of the middle (*otitis media*) or outer ear canal (*otitis externa*). Mullein and St John's wort infused oil are the traditional herbs used to ease inflammation, pain and infection. Place a couple of drops (1 drop for children) onto the outer ear and massage gently (i.e. not into the ear hole, but around the area). Alternatively, use compresses of the external herbs below. Herbal infusions of mullein can also be taken. To help the body fight the infection, internal immune support is needed, and echinacea and elderberry in infusions, tinctures or syrups can be taken; see page 74 for immune support guidance and page 140 for children.

INTERNAL HERBS *Echinacea, elderberry, garlic, St John's wort, mullein, chamomile*

EXTERNAL HERBS *St John's wort, mullein, garlic, lavender, chamomile*

RECIPES *Steam inhalation (page 19); Immune tincture (page 80); Cough syrup/drops (pages 112, 115); Garlic & mullein oil (page 140)*

Seasonal hayfever is caused by an allergy to pollen, which causes inflammation of the upper respiratory tract (nose, throat, sinuses) and sometimes eyes. Irritation, itchiness and over-production of mucus can be eased herbally by using an infusion or tincture of a mix of the herbs below. Herbalists believe that the key to helping hayfever symptoms is to start taking anti-allergy herbs early, before the 'season' starts, therefore if you have symptoms in June, try to take herbs in April and May. Allergic rhinitis, which produces similar symptoms, is also an allergic response but can be caused by other allergens such as animal fur and dust, which can be treated in the same way as hayfever. Itchy, irritated eyes can be soothed using cotton pads soaked with chilled infusions of chamomile and eyebright and placed over closed eyes.

INTERNAL HERBS *Nettle, elderflower, eyebright, plantain, chamomile, ground ivy*

RECIPES *Anti-allergy infusion (see below), Itchy-eye cooler cubes (page 118); Nasal wash (page 121)*

Anti-allergy infusion

This herbal mix combines elderflower, plantain and nettle to help reduce the inflammatory allergic reaction in hayfever and to soothe itchy insect bites and stings. These herbs have been used for their soothing effects and can help calm hot, irritated membranes of the nose, throat and eyes.

20g (¾ oz) dried plantain
20g (¾ oz) dried nettle leaves
20g (¾ oz) dried chamomile flowers
20g (¾ oz) dried eyebright

Combine the herbs and store in a labelled and dated airtight container.

TO USE Infuse 2 teaspoons of the herbal mix in 200ml (⅓ pint) boiling water, cover and allow to steep for 10–15 minutes before drinking. Repeat up to 3 times a day.

SHELF LIFE Up to 1 year in a cool, dark place.

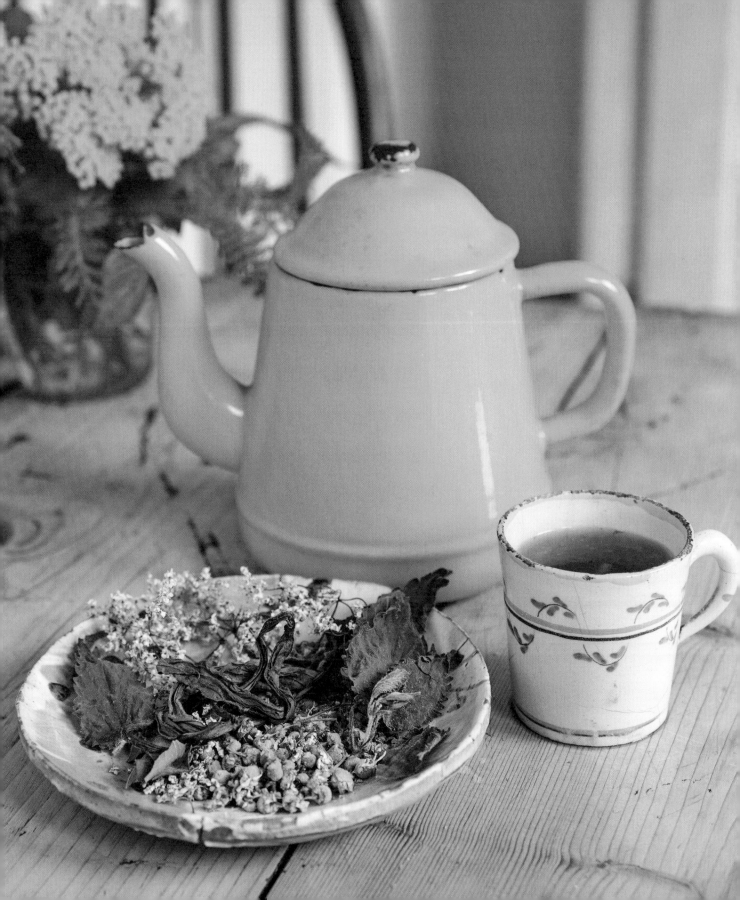

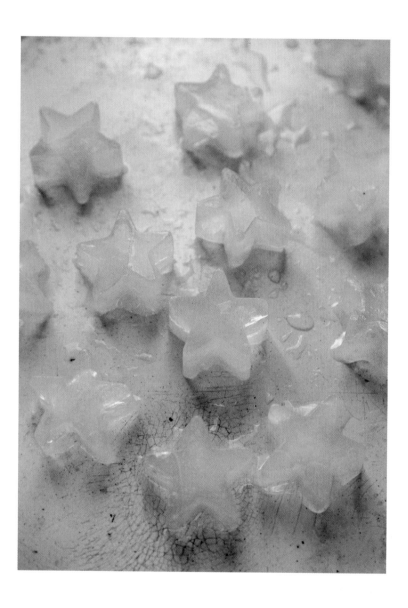

Itchy-eye cooler cubes

This recipe includes eyebright, a herb recorded as far back as the Ancient Greeks for its use in strengthening eyes and reducing inflammation. Combined with anti-inflammatory chamomile and elderflower, it makes a soothing remedy for puffy, itchy eyes caused by allergies. Perfect for hayfever, but it can also be used to help soothe strained and tired eyes.

1 teaspoon fresh or dried chamomile flowers
1 teaspoon fresh or dried eyebright
1 teaspoon fresh or dried elderflowers
100ml (3½ fl oz) boiling water
50ml (2 fl oz) witch hazel water (optional)

Place the fresh or dried herbs in a bowl or cup and cover with the boiling water. Allow to infuse until cool.

Strain out and discard the herbs, retaining the liquid. Combine the liquid with the witch hazel water, if using. Either use the liquid straightaway for the eye area (see below) or freeze in ice-cube trays.

TO USE Soak cotton wool pads in the chilled infusion and place over closed eyelids, sit back and relax for 10–15 minutes. For the frozen version, take an ice cube and wrap it in a layer of muslin or kitchen towel, then pat gently around the eye area to cool and soothe. Repeat as needed.

SHELF LIFE The chilled mixture will keep for up to 2 days in the fridge. The ice cubes will keep for up to 1 year in an airtight container in the freezer.

SORE THROAT

Swelling, irritation and pain in the throat is usually associated with colds and flu (page 108) and occasionally hayfever (page 116). For bacterial and tonsillitis infections, seek advice from a healthcare practitioner.

INTERNAL HERBS *Echinacea, elderberry, sage, blackberry, honeysuckle, clove, thyme, ground ivy*

RECIPES *Immune tincture (page 80); Elderberry pastilles (page 81); Fire cider (page 82); Cold & flu infusion (page 108); Elderberry syrup (page 111); Sore throat gargle (see right); Cough drops (page 115); Ginger & honey throat melts (page 120);*

Sore throat gargle

Echinacea angustifolia and clove help to numb pain. The honey and marshmallow soothe and coat the throat, while the sage is traditionally used to tighten and cool hot, irritated membranes. The elderberry helps fight viral infection and boosts the immune system. All these tinctures can be made or bought from good herbal suppliers.

20ml (4 teaspoons) echinacea angustifolia tincture
10ml (2 teaspoons) marshmallow tincture
10ml (2 teaspoons) sage tincture
10ml (2 teaspoons) elderberry tincture
10ml (2 teaspoons) clove or cardamom tincture or hydrosol
10ml (2 teaspoons) honey (optional)

Place all the ingredients in a glass bottle and shake to combine. Label and date the bottle.

TO USE Shake the bottle well to mix the ingredients thoroughly each time. Place 1–2 teaspoons of the mixture in a small cup with 1 tablespoon of water. Use as a gargle. Spit out or swallow as you prefer. Repeat as necessary up to 4 times a day.

SHELF LIFE Up to 1 year in a cool, dark place.

TIP Place the mixture in a spray bottle for an easy-to-use remedy. Simply spray a couple of times at the back of the throat.

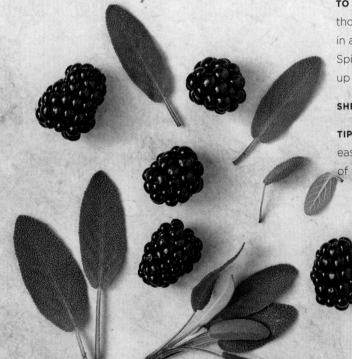

Ginger & honey throat melts

This quick and easy recipe makes a soothing remedy for coating and soothing sore, inflamed throats. The marshmallow root and slippery elm contains anti-inflammatory mucilages that line the throat, and the honey, ginger and clove bring warming, pain-relieving properties. These will also make a simple remedy for mild constipation. Suck a couple and you should see relief within a few hours.

3 tablespoons room-temperature unrefined
   coconut oil (ideally soft, but not melted)
1 teaspoon marshmallow root or slippery
   elm powder
1 teaspoon honey
¼ teaspoon ground ginger
¼ teaspoon ground cloves

In a bowl, stir all the ingredients together to combine well. Pour into an ice cube tray, ideally with small, rounded divisions suitable for making suckable lozenges. This should make about 8–10 melts. Place in the freezer to set. Once set, these can be placed in an airtight container and stored in the freezer.

TO USE Suck one of the melts as needed. These are high in calories, so do not exceed 3–4 per day.

SHELF LIFE In the freezer for up to a year.

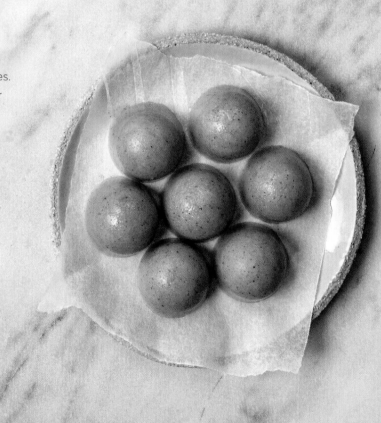

SINUSITIS

Bacterial or viral infection of the sinus cavities around the eyes and nose can cause an overproduction of mucus, congestion and a pain similar to a frontal headache. An associated symptom includes an increase in pain when bending forwards. Steam inhalations with decongestant and antibacterial essential oils can help to ease breathing and congestion (page 19), while the Anti-allergy infusion recipe (page 116) can give symptomatic relief and dry up mucus. Also see the Immune health section (page 74) for remedies that help the body fight any underlying infection. Ground ivy and plantain are 'specific' traditional herbs taken in infusions or as tinctures for sinus problems, and thyme adds an extra antibacterial boost to help with infection.

INTERNAL HERBS *Ground ivy, plantain, elderflower, echinacea, marshmallow, garlic, eyebright*

EXTERNAL HERBS *(in steam inhalations or facial compresses): Thyme, sage, rosemary, eucalyptus, peppermint, lavender*

ESSENTIAL OILS *(in steam inhalations): Thyme, eucalyptus, tea tree, rosemary, peppermint, sweet birch, lavender, frankincense*

RECIPES *Immune tincture (page 80); Elderberry pastilles (page 81); Cold & flu infusion (page 108); Elderberry syrup (page 111); Anti-allergy infusion (page 116); Nasal wash (see right)*

Nasal wash

Neti pots (see below) have traditionally been used in Ayurvedic medicine to ease nasal congestion and infection and can be helpful in some cases of sinusitis and hayfever. They help to 'wash' out excess mucus and irritants, if the cause is due to pollen or dust, for example. Saline water is commonly used, but adding a mild infusion of herbs can add an extra healing boost.

¼ teaspoon chopped fresh or dried ground ivy
¼ teaspoon chopped fresh or dried plantain
¼ teaspoon chopped fresh or dried thyme
250ml (9 fl oz) boiling filtered water
¼ teaspoon salt
¼ teaspoon bicarbonate of soda

Place the herbs in a mug and pour over the boiling water. Leave to infuse for 5 minutes, then strain and discard the solids.

Pour the strained liquid into a neti pot and add the salt and bicarbonate of soda. Mix well.

TO USE You will need a neti pot, which is a long-spouted jug easily found online and in healthcare shops. Stand over a sink. Tilting the head to one side, pour half the liquid slowly through the upper nostril and allow it to flow out of the lower nostril. You may need to blow your nose gently afterwards to remove any excess. Repeat on the other side. Only for adults and children over 12 years old. Not to be used frequently.

SHELF LIFE Use immediately.

SKIN, HAIR & NAILS
ACNE

Acne is particularly associated with adolescents and hormonal conditions such as PMS/PMT. Therefore, investigating hormonal, dietary and digestive issues may help to remove underlying causes. Herbally, bitter herbs that support proper digestion and elimination of waste in the body, and herbal infusions that support the tissue-clearing lymph system help towards clearing the skin. Dip a flannel in a herbal infusion made from any of the external herbs below and place over the face for a few minutes to open and clean out the pores, then splash with cold water or witch hazel to tone the skin. Weekly facial steams are also beneficial to clear congested, spotty skin (page 19). If a big spot threatens to come out overnight, a drop of lavender essential oil on the spot before bed can reduce its redness. Try the light, non-oily nourishing skin cream to soothe and calm outbreaks.

INTERNAL HERBS *Calendula, cleavers, red clover, nettle, burdock, dandelion, curly dock, echinacea*

EXTERNAL HERBS *Calendula, lavender, rose, eucalyptus, gotu kola, echinacea, tea tree, aloe vera, witch hazel*

RECIPES *Bitter digestive spray (page 66); Skin beauty tea (page 126); Spot-banishing gel (right); Nourishing skin cream (opposite); Floral face toner (page 131)*

Spot-banishing gel

Use this antibacterial spot gel overnight to fight infection and calm redness. Fresh aloe vera gel can be used, but it will not last as long as the prepared, shop-bought type from a tube.

50ml (2 fl oz) aloe vera gel
5 drops thyme essential oil
10 drops lavender essential oil
10 drops lemon essential oil

Whisk the essential oils into the aloe vera drop by drop until well combined. Store in a pump-top bottle or small tin and apply with a clean cotton bud.

TO USE Dab onto spots as needed.

SHELF LIFE Up to 6 months in a cool, dark place.

Nourishing skin cream

This cream is easy to whip up and can be adapted using the ingredients below to create your own bespoke product for the face or body, tailored to your skin's needs. Aloe vera gel is needed as the leaf gel is not suitable for this recipe.

50ml (2 fl oz) aloe vera gel
5–10ml (1–2 teaspoons) base oil
5ml (1 teaspoon) booster
10–20 drops essential oil

ACNE/OILY SKIN

Base oils: yarrow or calendula infused
   grapeseed or jojoba oil
Booster: willow bark tincture or witch hazel water
Essential oils: lemon, tea tree, lavender, yarrow,
   chamomile blue

ANTI-AGEING/DRY SKIN

Base oils: calendula, marshmallow and/or
   gotu kola infused almond oil, cold-pressed
   sunflower oil
Booster: rosehip, macadamia, wheatgerm, hemp oil
Essential oils: frankincense, myrrh, rose, neroli

ECZEMA

Base oils: calendula or chickweed infused oil
Booster: chamomile floral water
Essential oils: chamomile blue, lavender, yarrow

PSORIASIS

Base oils: chamomile or chickweed infused oil
Booster: evening primrose oil, liquorice tincture,
   turmeric tincture, evening primrose oil
Essential oil: lavender

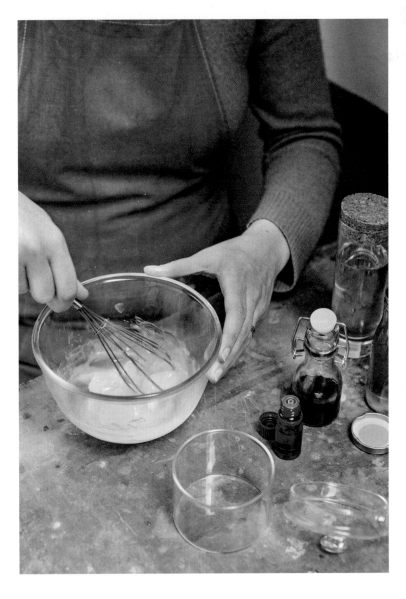

Whisk the base oils into the aloe vera drop by drop until well combined. It's imporatant to do this stage slowly to keep a serum consistency. Next, whisk in the booster and essential oils thoroughly. Keep in a pump-top bottle or tin, label and date.

TO USE Apply twice daily, or as required.

SHELF LIFE Up to 6 months in a cool, dark place.

BOILS & ABSCESSES

Boils are hot, painful, pus-filled spots caused by infections in the top layers of skin around a hair follicle. Abscesses are deeper infections of the skin's layers. For either problem, boosting the body's immune system will help battle the infection. Herbs that are bitter or support the lymph system (the liquid in tissues that washes out impurities and moves infection to the lymph nodes) help support the skin's ability to eliminate toxins and heal. Drink an infusion of lymphatic herbs or take bitter herbs as suggested on page 66 to help. Burdock is a traditional deep skin healer and a specific herb for boils. Warm compresses using herbs listed in the external herbs section below can help to draw infection to the surface of the skin, helping to clear the infection.

CAUTION Cellulitis is a more serious condition characterised by pain and inflammation, with tightness and redness of the skin, sometimes with fever where the deeper tissues are infected over a larger area. If suspected, this should be seen by a doctor.

INTERNAL HERBS *Calendula, echinacea, cleavers, nettle, red clover, dandelion, plantain, elderberry, burdock, curly dock*

EXTERNAL HERBS *Calendula, gotu kola, tea tree, thyme, plantain, marshmallow leaf or root*

RECIPES *Herbal compresses and poultices (page 20); Healing ointment (page 38); Drawing ointment (right)*

Drawing ointment

Drawing ointments help to 'draw' out splinters from the skin, and pus from spots, boils and abscesses, bringing them to a head and helping them to heal.

20g (¾ oz) marshmallow root powder or
    slippery elm powder
20g (¾ oz) bentonite clay
1 teaspoon honey
5 drops essential oil (choose from tea tree, eucalyptus,
    yarrow, lavender)
30–50ml (1–2 fl oz) strong herbal infusion (choose from
    calendula, plantain or yarrow)

Place the powder and clay in a bowl. Add the honey and essential oil drops and just enough of the infusion while it is still warm to create a thick, paste-like consistency.

TO USE Apply a little of the paste to the affected area and secure with a plaster or bandage. Leave in place for a few hours, refreshing with new paste and fresh dressing as necessary.

SHELF LIFE Store in the fridge in an airtight container and use within 3 days.

IMPETIGO

WARTS & VERRUCAS

This skin infection is caused by the streptococcus bacteria. It is most commonly found in children, around the nose, mouth and hands, but can also appear elsewhere. The persistent red sores are classed in two ways: non-bullous (scaly, non-weeping) and bullous (weeping, forming golden crusts around the lesions and highly contagious). Ensure strict hygiene measures are followed, such as using separate washcloths, towels and bedding, which should be washed after each use on a hot setting. Internal immune-supporting herbs are needed (page 74). Wound-healing herbs can also be made into infusions, which once cooled can be used as compresses to aid healing. Impetigo can be persistent, and if there is no change, antibiotics may be needed as well.

INTERNAL HERBS *Echinacea, calendula, curly dock, burdock, cleavers*

EXTERNAL HERBS *Calendula, thyme, myrrh, eucalyptus*

ESSENTIAL OILS *Myrrh, eucalyptus, tea tree, thyme*

These common skin protrusions are caused by the human papilloma virus (HPV), which is usually picked up through a cut in the skin, most frequently in moist places such as swimming pools and shared showers. Both are infectious and need to be combatted by boosting the body's immune system with both internal and topical immune-boosting and antiviral herbs. Traditionally, the juice of garlic, fresh latex of dandelion or greater celandine has been painted on the wart and covered with a plaster to reduce growth. Take care not to get greater celandine on healthy skin as it can be slightly caustic. Warts and verrucas tend to heal on their own accord but can take years, so treatment requires perseverance.

INTERNAL HERBS *Echinacea, elderberry, eucalyptus, thyme*

EXTERNAL HERBS *Dandelion, greater celandine, St John's wort, melissa, thyme, eucalyptus, garlic*

ESSENTIAL OILS *Eucalyptus, tea tree, thyme*

RECIPE *Immune tincture (page 80)*

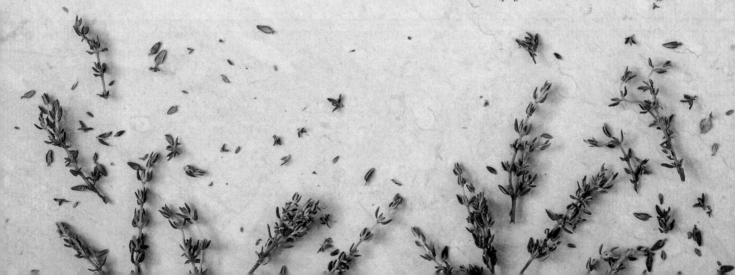

ECZEMA

This chronic condition has complex origins and can be caused by external irritants, but also as a result of immune dysfunction, hormonal imbalances and a range of allergies both external and dietary. Herbalists treat eczema through balancing the body's overactive immune system and improving digestion. Supporting the digestive system is essential for proper absorption of nutrients and elimination of waste from the body, both of which affect skin function. Bitter herb tinctures and skin-clearing herbal infusions (page 66) can be taken to support this. Externally, bathing with porridge oats tied in a piece of muslin to cleanse, soothe and protect the skin is an effective remedy. Itchy rashes can be soothed with fresh chickweed juice. For stubborn eczema, where home treatment has not helped, seek guidance from a local herbalist.

INTERNAL HERBS *Calendula, burdock, cleavers, nettle, red clover, curly dock, horsetail, mahonia, dandelion, gotu kola, milk thistle*

EXTERNAL HERBS *Oats, chamomile, lavender, calendula, chickweed, plantain*

RECIPES *Healing ointment (page 38) Skin beauty tea (right); Bitter drops (page 66); Immune tincture (page 80); Nourishing skin cream (page 123); Oaty bath balls (page 129)*

Skin beauty tea

The herbs below are used by herbalists for their skin-clearing properties. Cleavers, nettles, red clover and calendula are diuretic and traditionally used as 'lymphatic' herbs that cleanse and clear the tissues, and in turn, the skin. Milk thistle seed is used to support the liver function and aid the removal of waste from the body.

20g (¾ oz) dried cleavers
20g (¾ oz) dried nettle leaves
20g (¾ oz) dried dandelion leaves
20g (¾ oz) dried red clover flowers
20g (¾ oz) dried calendula petals
20g (¾ oz) ground milk thistle seed

Mix the above ingredients in a bowl, then store in an airtight container marked with a label and date.

TO USE Use 2 teaspoons of the mixture in a cup of boiling water. Cover and allow to infuse for 10–15 minutes. Drink up to 3 cups a day.

SHELF LIFE Up to 1 year in a cool, dark place.

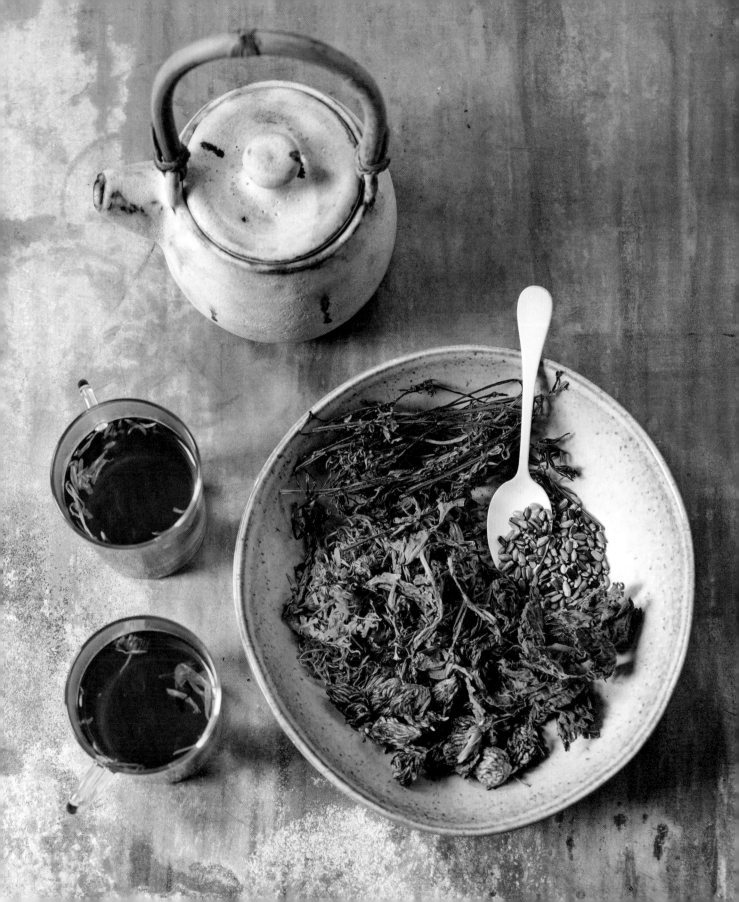

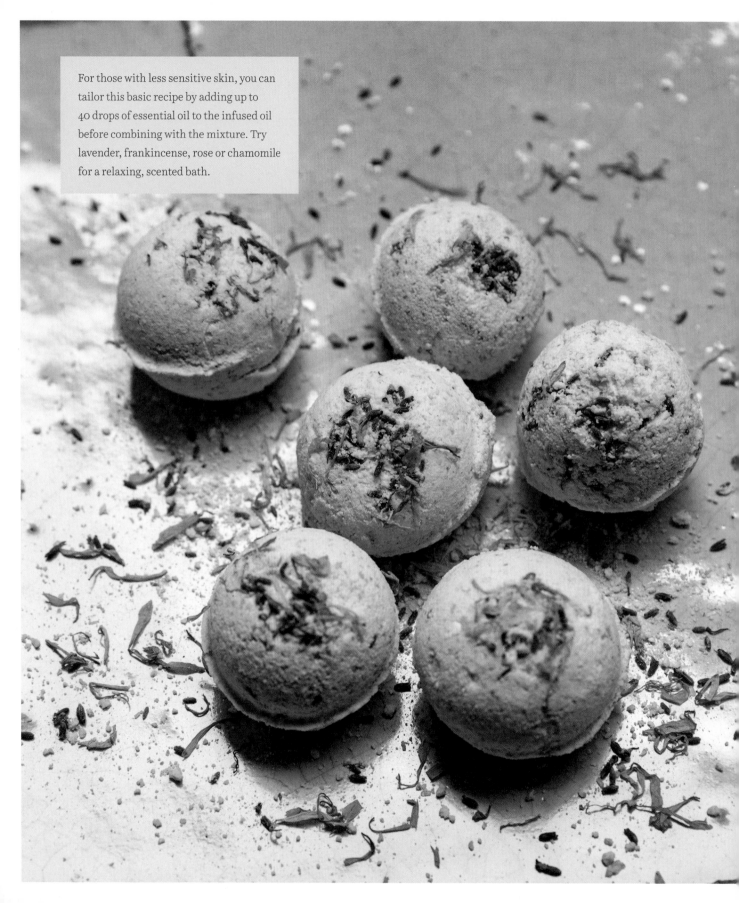

For those with less sensitive skin, you can tailor this basic recipe by adding up to 40 drops of essential oil to the infused oil before combining with the mixture. Try lavender, frankincense, rose or chamomile for a relaxing, scented bath.

Oaty bath balls

These skin-calming bath bombs contain gentle, nourishing milky oats, anti-inflammatory chamomile, anti-itch chickweed and soothing salts. Ideal for eczema, itchy skin as well as a nourishing, luxury skin soak.

130g (4½ oz) bicarbonate of soda
125g (4½ oz) sea salt or Epsom salts
65g (2¼ oz) citric acid
25g (1oz) ground oats
2 tablespoons each of dried lavender
 and calendula flowers
10ml (2 teaspoons) chickweed infused oil
15ml (½ fl oz) chamomile decoction
cornflour, to coat the moulds

Mix all the dry ingredients, including the herbs, together in a bowl until well combined.

Gradually add the oil and decoction, mixing well with a fork until it takes on the consistency of damp sand. The mixture should hold together when squeezed; if not, add another ¼ teaspoon of decoction and oil until you reach the desired consistency.

Using cornflour, coat bath bomb moulds or a muffin tray, and press the mixture firmly into the moulds, then gently tap out and leave to dry on a baking tray for 24–48 hours until hard. Store in an airtight container.

TO USE Add 1 bomb to a bath, allow to fizzle, then sit back and relax.

SHELF LIFE Up to 6 months.

This condition is caused by an overproduction of skin cells, which presents as shiny patches often found on the scalp and around joints such as the knees and elbows. It is a complex and chronic condition, thought to be caused by an overactive immune system, hormonal imbalance or a range of allergies including dietary. Holistic treatment of psoriasis aims to balance the overactive immune system and remove any allergens in the diet or lifestyle that could be triggering the condition. Mahonia and milk thistle have been used by herbalists for their action on the liver to help clear stubborn skin conditions and for slowing down skin cell production in problem areas. Baths using anti-inflammatory herbal infusions and porridge oats in a sock to soothe and wash the skin can also help. Psoriasis can be a persistent problem, and is often best treated with guidance from a herbalist.

EXTERNAL HERBS *Calendula, burdock, mahonia, angelica, celery seed, cleavers, milk thistle, nettle, red clover, liquorice, oats*

RECIPES *Digestive bitters mix (page 66); Immune tincture (page 80); Nourishing skin cream (page 123); Skin beauty tea (page 126); Oaty bath balls (left)*

ITCHING/RASHES

RINGWORM

Itchy skin and rashes caused by a temporary irritation can be treated with simple herbal washes or compresses using porridge oats, fresh chickweed or other soothing herbs (see external herbs below). Porridge oats in a muslin cloth, soaked in hot water then cooled, can also be used as a gentle, moisturising wash. For itchy rashes caused by allergies, eczema and chickenpox, please refer to the relevant sections.

INTERNAL HERBS *Nettle, plantain, chamomile*

EXTERNAL HERBS *Chickweed, chamomile, lavender, aloe vera gel, oats, calendula*

RECIPES *Nourishing skin cream (page 123); Oaty bath balls (page 129)*

Ringworm is an itchy skin infection caused by a fungus rather than a 'worm' and appears as silver or red patches delineated with a red outline. It should not be confused with a bullseye ring mark after a tick bite, which may suggest Lyme's disease and will require medical treatment. For ringworm, boost the body's immunity using tips from the Immune health section (page 74), and use antifungal herbs in washes, compresses and creams with added antifungal essential oils.

INTERNAL HERBS *Echinacea, sage, thyme, oregano*

EXTERNAL HERBS *Thyme, oregano, calendula*

ESSENTIAL OILS *Thyme, tea tree, eucalyptus, oregano, myrrh*

RECIPE *Antifungal powder (page 146)*

> ## STRETCH MARKS
> See page 160 for more on this, and the Supple skin balm recipe, which doubles as our go-to recipe for improving general skin elasticity.

WRINKLES

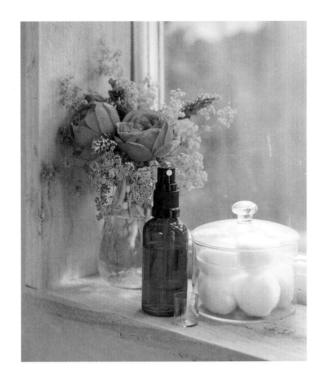

We should learn to love our wrinkles – after all, they chart our lives and give our faces their unique character. Radiant skin can be achieved by anyone, simply by living a healthy and balanced lifestyle full of good nutrition and herbs to support healthy tissues and the body's digestive system, which helps to eliminate wastes. Astringent herbs, such as lady's mantle and rose, have been traditionally used to tighten and tone skin, along with herbs such as marshmallow and calendula to moisturise and protect. Use these herbs in face washes, floral water toners, or in nourishing, anti-ageing creams.

INTERNAL HERBS *Red clover, nettle, calendula, cleavers, horsetail, borage seed oil, evening primrose oil*

EXTERNAL HERBS *Calendula, lady's mantle, rose, rosehip seed oil, elderflower*

ESSENTIAL OILS *Frankincense, rose, lavender*

RECIPES *Nourishing skin cream (page 123); Floral face toner (right)*

Floral face toner

Elderflowers help brighten and even skin tone, while lady's mantle has been valued for its skin-tightening properties throughout the centuries. Combined with gently toning anti-inflammatory rose petals, this toner will leave the skin soft, cleansed and radiant. Follow with the Nourishing skin cream on page 123 for adding moisture. The hydrosol versions of these herbs also make a beautiful scented toner.

1 teaspoon fresh or dried elderflowers
1 teaspoon fresh or dried lady's mantle
1 teaspoon fresh or dried rose petals

Place the herbs in a mug of boiling water and allow to infuse until cool. Strain and discard the solids.

TO USE Using cotton wool pads or a soft cloth, wipe the face with the mixture after cleansing twice daily. Alternatively, store in a spray bottle and spritz the face. Follow with a moisturiser.

SHELF LIFE Store in the fridge for up to 3 days.

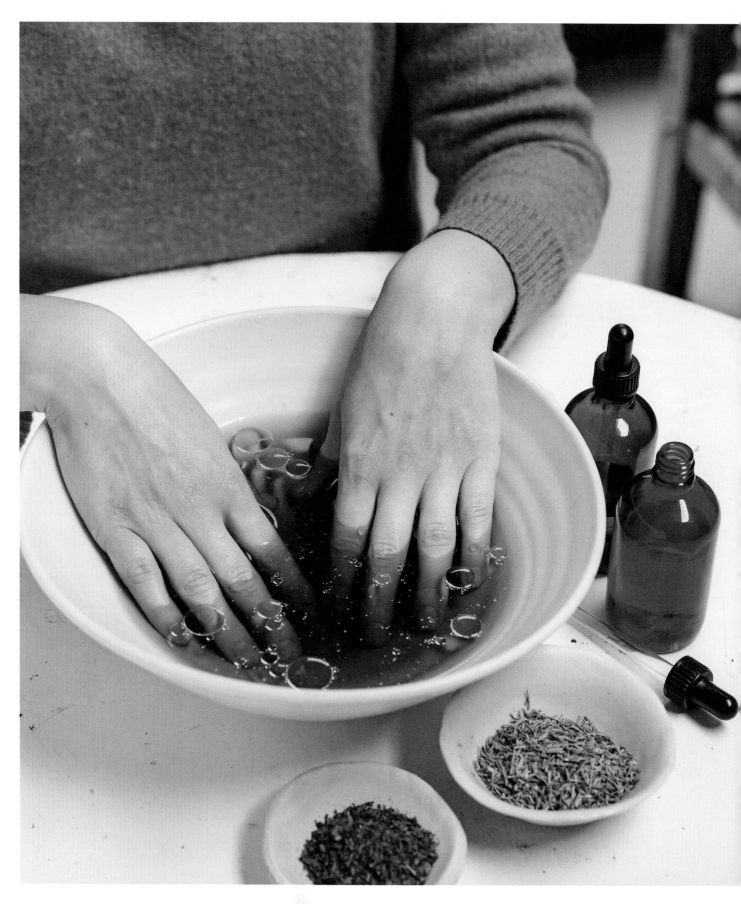

WEAK NAILS

Nettle and horsetail contain silica and other minerals that help strengthen weak nails, and can be drunk in herbal infusions and used for hand baths. Flaking, fragile nails may be caused by long-term use of nail varnishes and chemicals such as household cleaners. Weak nails may also signify a nutritional deficiency, poor circulation or other underlying conditions, such as Reynaud syndrome, which might need medical investigation.

Nail-strengthening hand bath

1 litre (1¾ pint) water
2 tablespoons fresh or 1 tablespoon dried nettle leaves
2 tablespoons fresh or 1 tablespoon dried horsetail
2 drops lavender, lemon or frankincense essential oil
½ teaspoon carrier oil, such as sunflower or olive oil

Place the water and herbs together in a pan and bring to a simmer for 5 minutes before turning off the heat. Cover and allow to infuse until the infusion has reached skin temperature. Strain the liquid into a bowl.

Add the essential oils to the carrier oil and mix well, then add to the liquid in the bowl.

TO USE Find somewhere comfortable to sit where you can place the bowl within hand's reach. Soak your varnish-free nails (and hands if you wish) for 10–15 minutes. Remove from the bowl and massage in the oils that will have coated the skin and nails. Repeat twice a week.

SHELF LIFE Use immediately.

Athlete's foot and fungal nail infections can be treated by supporting the immune system internally to help fight off infection. Use infusions of antifungal herbs in foot and hand baths, along with creams or powders using essential oils. The antifungal Four thieves vinegar (page 85) can be diluted and used in foot soaks, or use the Antifungal powder as a drying 'talcum' powder (page 146). For fungal nails, carefully paint the nail with tea tree or eucalyptus essential oils (diluted if using on children).

INTERNAL HERBS *Echinacea, elderberry, thyme, oregano, eucalyptus, pau d'arco, burdock*

EXTERNAL HERBS *Oregano, thyme, calendula, sage, rosemary, myrrh*

ESSENTIAL OILS *Thyme, oregano, eucalyptus, tea tree, myrrh, lavender*

RECIPES *Immune tincture (page 80); Four thieves vinegar (page 85); Antifungal powder (page 146)*

FOOT HEALTH

HAIR

Aches, hard skin, corns, athlete's foot – many of us are on our feet most of the day so no wonder they feel a little under pressure and build up tough, protective skin. For hard skin and corns, or just as a relaxing treat, try a foot soak using the following herbs infused with an added handful of sea salts to soften and soothe. Soak the feet for 20–30 minutes, then gently buff away hard areas of skin. A regular cream or carrier oil with added lavender, lemon, tea tree or eucalyptus essential oils can be massaged into the skin to moisturise and protect. For fungal infections, see Athlete's foot and fungal nails section (page 133).

EXTERNAL HERBS *Calendula, yarrow, eucalyptus, nettle, peppermint*

There are plenty of herbs traditionally used for strengthening and adding shine to healthy hair, including those high in silica such as nettle and horsetail. Rosemary helps to stimulate scalp circulation and hair growth and can be taken internally or used in hair rinses. For hair loss it is best to understand the underlying complaint, which may be nutritional, genetic or due to a hormonal imbalance such as thyroid dysfunction and may need guidance from a healthcare practitioner. For male baldness, try the advice on page 145.

INTERNAL HERBS *Nettle, rosemary*

EXTERNAL HERBS *Rosemary, sage, nettle, horsetail*

RECIPES *Herbal hair rinse (opposite); Castor oil hair-conditioning mask (page 137)*

HAIR BOOSTER HERBS

FOR DARK HAIR
2 tablespoons fresh
    or 1 tablespoon dried
    rosemary, chopped
2 tablespoons fresh or
    1 tablespoon dried
    sage, chopped

FOR BLONDE HAIR
2 tablespoons fresh
    or 1 tablespoon dried
    chamomile flowers
1 tablespoon lemon juice
7.5cm/3 in strip of
    lemon peel

FOR RED HAIR
2 tablespoons fresh
    or 1 tablespoon dried
    calendula flowers
2 tablespoons rooibos
    tea leaves or dried
    hibiscus flowers
    (or both)

FOR DANDRUFF
2 tablespoons fresh
    aromatic herbs such
    as rosemary, sage,
    oregano or thyme,
    chopped

Herbal hair rinse

Nettle, rosemary and sage stimulate and nourish the scalp to help healthy hair growth. The horsetail and nettle also contain silica, which is thought to help boost hair and skin quality.

BASE HAIR RINSE INGREDIENTS
2 tablespoons fresh or 1 tablespoon
    dried nettle leaves, chopped
2 tablespoons fresh or 1 tablespoon
    dried horsetail, chopped
1 tablespoon apple cider vinegar
1 litre water
herbs of your choice from the hair
    booster box opposite (optional)

Make a simple decoction using your base hair rinse ingredients and your choice of herbs from the box. Place them in a pan, add the water, bring to a boil then simmer gently for 15 minutes. Remove from the heat and allow to cool.

   Strain and place in a jug to be used the same day.

TO USE Wash and rinse your hair using your normal shampoo and conditioner. Use the cooled herbal decoction as a final rinse, ensuring you massage it well into the scalp.

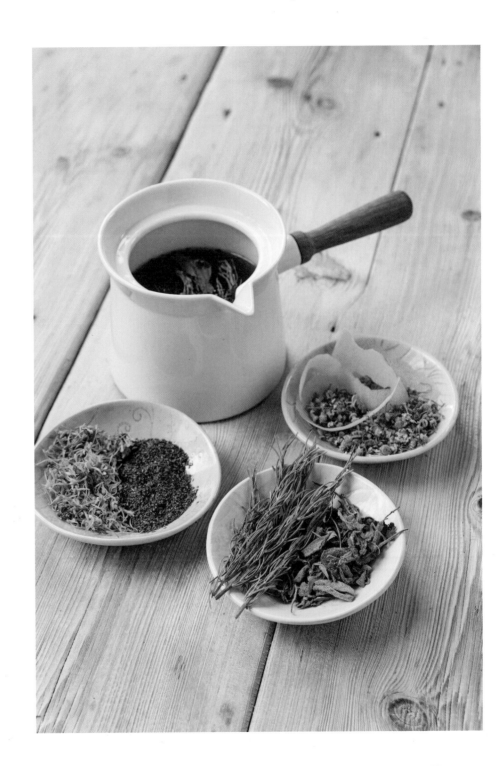

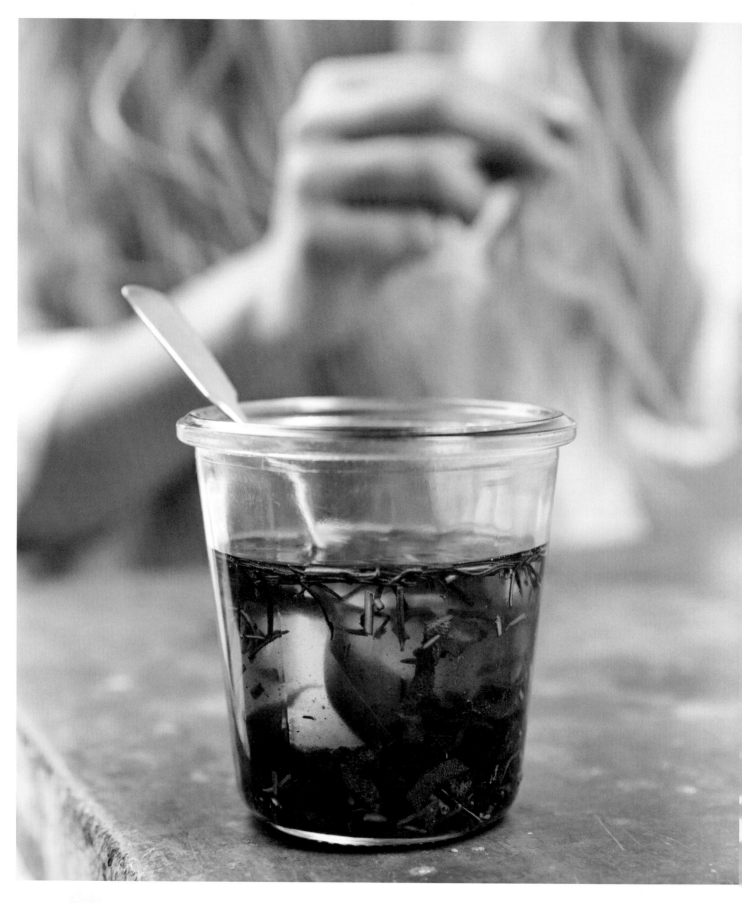

Castor oil hair-conditioning mask

This nourishing hair mask uses herbal infused castor oil to replenish and add shine. To add vibrance for different hair types, choose a bespoke blend from below.

75ml (2½ fl oz) castor oil
75ml (2½ fl oz) olive oil

FOR DARK HAIR
2 tablespoons dried rosemary
2 tablespoons dried sage
20 drops rosemary essential oil

FOR BLONDE HAIR
2 tablespoons dried chamomile flowers
2 tablespoons dried citrus peel
20 drops lemon essential oil

FOR RED HAIR
2 tablespoons dried calendula flowers
2 tablespoons rooibos tea leaves
20 drops peppermint essential oil

Crush the dried herbs and place into a jar. Cover with the castor and olive oil and infuse for 4 hours in a bain-marie (page 24). Strain out the herbs and reserve the oil, then add the essential oil and mix well. Bottle, label and date.

TO USE Apply enough infused oil to coat the hair from root to tip, massage into the scalp and brush through with a wide-toothed comb. Keep the mask on for at least 1 hour (overnight is even better). To wash off, massage a generous amount of shampoo into the oily hair without water. Once the shampoo is worked in, wash out with warm water. Repeat the wash with more shampoo to remove all of the surface oil.

NOTE Before use, test some of this product on a small section of hair overnight, particularly if you use hair colourants.

Dandruff is a flaky skin condition of the scalp (and sometimes eyebrows), usually caused by a fungal infection. After shampooing, use the hair rinse on page 135 or a tablespoon of nettle-infused vinegar added to a litre of water for a final rinse. You can also add a tablespoon of nettle tincture and some antifungal essential oils to your shampoo using the selection below.

INTERNAL HERBS *Echinacea, nettle, rosemary, sage, oregano, thyme, burdock*

EXTERNAL HERBS *Nettle, rosemary, sage, oregano, thyme*

ESSENTIAL OILS *Eucalyptus, tea tree, lavender, thyme, oregano*

CHILDREN'S HEALTH

CHICKENPOX

DOSAGE FOR CHILDREN

When giving a new herb to a child for the first time, give a small amount and observe carefully for any symptoms or reactions. Below is a rough guide to dosages for children:

BABIES AGED 6 MONTHS-2 YEARS 10% of adult dose (consult a herbalist when giving herbs to children under 2 years old)

CHILDREN AGED 2-6 YEARS 10–30% of adult dose

CHILDREN AGED 6-10 YEARS 30–50% of adult dose

CHILDREN AGED 6-14 YEARS 50–80% of adult dose

CHILDREN AGED OVER 14 80–100% of adult dose

Not all herbs are suitable for children.
Here's a list of some that can be used:

Chamomile, echinacea, elderflower, elderberry, rose, lavender, linden blossom, hawthorn, peppermint, plantain, lemon balm, oats, daisy, cleavers, calendula, mullein, honeysuckle, poppy, dandelion, nettle, violet, wild cherry, self-heal, culinary herbs (see pages 28–33).

A highly infectious childhood illness, chickenpox is caused by the varicella-zoster virus and characterised by an itchy red rash of small, blister-like spots that can occur anywhere on the body. Symptoms tend to last 7–10 days in children and are usually mild, causing a slight fever and irritability. Most people develop immunity after contracting the virus, but it can occur twice in some individuals. Chickenpox can also occur in adults, which is uncommon, however symptoms can be more severe.

The main focus for treatment is to lessen itching to prevent scarring from scratching. The infection is usually self-limiting, but you can support the immune system with herbs and diet to shorten the duration, severity and help lessen the chance of secondary infection. A soothing tea from any of the internal herbs below can help comfort and encourage sleep in uncomfortable and irritated patients. To ease scratching, a warm herbal bath with anti-inflammatory herbs such as chamomile, chickweed, calendula and soothing milky oats can also help.

INTERNAL HERBS *Lemon balm, catnip, chamomile, elderflower, oatstraw, linden flower, echinacea, elderberry*

EXTERNAL HERBS *Chickweed, lavender, linden flower, calendula, chamomile, oats*

RECIPES *Elderberry pastilles (page 81); Elderberry syrup (page 111); Oaty bath balls (page 129); Calamine lotion (opposite); Elder & linden flower infusion (page 142)*

COLIC
See page 166.

CONJUNCTIVITIS
See page 86.

Calamine lotion

This lotion can be used for most itchy skin conditions, including eczema, nappy rash and chickenpox.

4 teaspoons non-nano zinc oxide
2 teaspoons bicarbonate of soda
4 teaspoons pink clay
½ teaspoon glycerine
60ml (2 fl oz) strong chamomile infusion
   or witch hazel water or a mix of both
5 drops chamomile blue essential oil
10 drops lavender essential oil

In a bowl, mix together the zinc oxide, bicarbonate of soda and pink clay, breaking up any clumps with the back of a spoon.

In a separate bowl, dissolve the glycerine in the chamomile infusion or witch hazel.

Stir the liquid mix into the powders until fully combined. Add the essential oils and mix again. Spoon the lotion into a jar, label and date.

TO USE Apply to sore or irritated areas of skin as required. This lotion may leave marks on clothes, so apply with care.

SHELF LIFE Up to 2 months in the fridge.

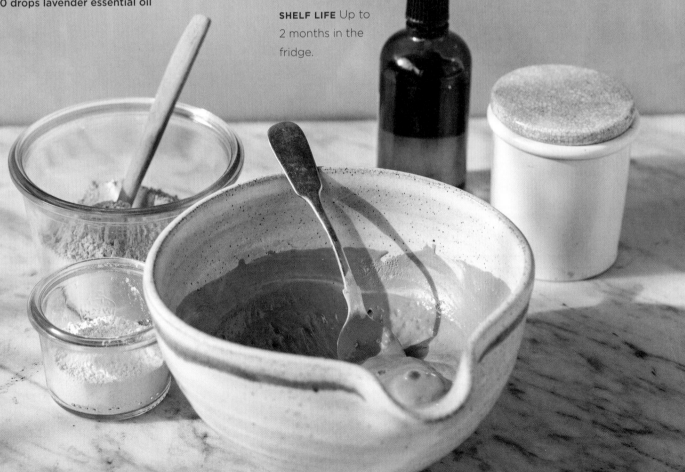

EARACHE

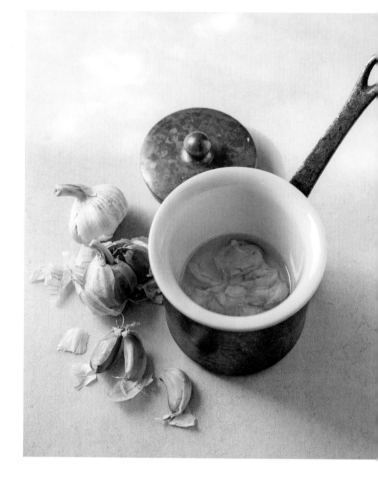

Earache can be a particularly common infection during the childhood years. It is caused by a bacterial or viral infection leading to painful inflammation and a build-up of fluid/pressure in the ear canal. Make a strong infusion of mullein, chamomile or yarrow, leave to cool to slightly warmer than body temperature, soak a small piece of cotton in the infusion and place in the ear.

To alleviate pain and congestion, massage behind and around the ear with 2 drops of lavender essential oil diluted in a teaspoon of carrier oil. Immune-boosting herbs taken in teas and syrups may help shorten the duration of the infection. Discharge from the ear, and swelling and redness of the outer ear and boney area behind the ears, can indicate a more serious infection; if this happens, seek medical attention.

INTERNAL HERBS *Chamomile, echinacea, garlic, cleavers, elderberry*

EXTERNAL HERBS *Mullein oil, chamomile, yarrow, garlic, thyme, lavender*

RECIPES *Garlic and mullein ear oil (right); Immune tincture – page 80 (for children over 6 years of age – see dosage instructions on page 138)*

Garlic & mullein ear oil

A simple home remedy used to battle infection and reduce inflammation. If you don't have mullein to hand, simply use garlic. For children over 4 years old.

1 small clove of garlic
1 teaspoon dried mullein leaves, crumbled
20ml (4 teaspoons) olive oil

Crush the garlic clove and place it in a bowl with the mullein.

Pour over the olive oil and allow to infuse in a bain-marie (page 24) for 20 minutes.

TO USE Soak a small piece of cotton in the oil and place in the affected ear for at least 30 minutes, 2–4 times a day.

SHELF LIFE Up to 1 week in the fridge. Not for internal use.

TUMMY ACHE

Children's gut bacteria and immune systems are still developing and they are constantly being exposed to new environmental microbes. Other reasons for tummy aches include constipation and trapped wind. If you think your child is constipated, increase dietary fibre or try 1 teaspoon of slippery elm powder mixed into a glass of fruit juice. For tummy ache caused by trapped wind, try fennel or mint tea. For unexplained tummy ache, try chamomile as it is antispasmodic, dispels wind and is slightly antimicrobial. A massage oil made from diluting any of the oils below in a carrier oil rubbed over the tummy can also soothe tummy ache.

HERBS *Fennel, mint, chamomile, slippery elm*

ESSENTIAL OILS *Fennel, chamomile, lavender*

RECIPES *Psyllium gel (page 63); Fig & prune syrup (page 63); Ginger & honey throat melts (page 120); Baby massage oil (page 168)*

CROUP

A type of respiratory infection, usually caused by a virus that affects the airways, particularly the trachea. It's characterised by a hoarse, 'barking' cough. Fever and runny nose may be present. It's usually a mild infection, with symptoms that start to improve after two days. If they don't, fever becomes high or there is difficulty breathing, seek medical attention. Give lots of fluids to maintain hydration: herbal teas sweetened with honey or herbal cordials such as elderflower or elderberry.

INTERNAL HERBS *Elderberry, elderflower, echinacea, catnip, chamomile*

FEVER

Fever in children is usually caused by infection; it is the body's natural defence to combat disease, as a raised body temperature makes for an inhospitable environment for bacteria and viruses. However, body temperature can rise quite suddenly in children, and if it becomes too high (38°C+/100°F+) it can become dangerous. Diaphoretic herbs encourage sweating and dilate the small blood vessels near the skin's surface in order to release heat from the body. Try an infusion with one or more of the herbs below, sweetened with honey if taste is a problem. Keep fluid intake high to avoid dehydration.

CAUTION! Seek medical advice if: the baby is under 3 months old and has a temperature of 38°C (100°F) or higher; in babies of 3–6 months, if the fever exceeds 39°C (102°F); if the fever lasts for longer than 3 days; if a child has convulsions, is dehydrated and unable to take fluids, or if a rash develops, especially if it does not disappear when a glass is rolled over it.

INTERNAL HERBS *Linden flower, yarrow, chamomile, elderflower, peppermint, self-heal, catnip*

RECIPES *Oral rehydration salts (page 71); Herbal hot toddy (page 74); Elderberry pastilles (page 81); Elder & linden flower infusion (page 142)*

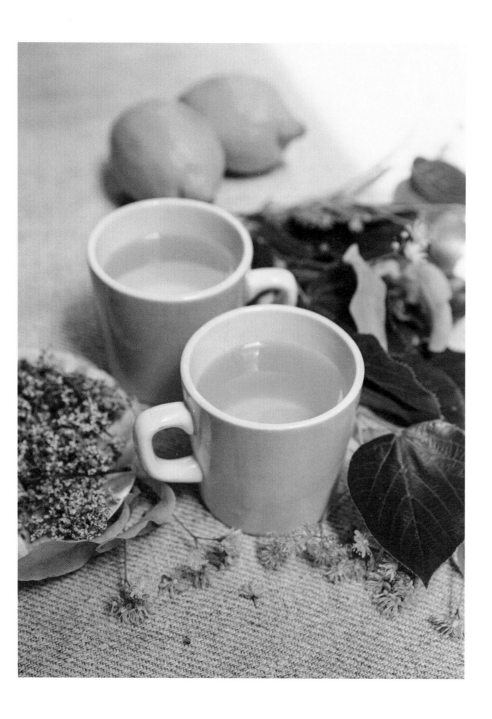

Elder & linden flower infusion

Elder and linden have both been used traditionally to bring down fever. Linden flower is a gentle herb, great for soothing irritated, young children and aiding restful sleep.

1 teaspoon fresh or dried elderflowers
1 teaspoon fresh or dried linden
  flowers
1 teaspoon honey (optional)

Place the herbs in a teapot or mug, pour over 3 cups of boiling water, cover with a lid or saucer, and allow to infuse for 5 minutes.

Strain, add honey, if using, and serve warm or cold.

TO USE 1 cup up to 3 times a day for children over 6 years of age.

HEADLICE

Headlice or 'nits' are visible, parasitic lice. Their eggs colonise the human head and spread through close contact, so these little pests are particularly common in primary-school children. Headlice feed on the blood of the scalp, making the skin very itchy, and their tiny egg capsules, known as nits, can often be seen clinging to the hairs. Regular washing and combing with a fine nit comb every four days can help to dislodge and kill the lice and eggs. Headlice do not like essential oils, so try adding a few drops of one of the oils below to your usual shampoo to discourage lice when there is an outbreak at school. Quassia chips can be made into a strong decoction (page 13), allowed to cool and poured over hair as a rinse to help kill headlice and deter re-infection.

EXTERNAL HERBS *Quassia wood, eucalyptus, neem oil*

ESSENTIAL OILS *(External use only) Cedarwood, lavender, tea tree, eucalyptus, rosemary*

Headlice oil treatment

This headlice oil uses insecticidal essential oils, which can kill resident lice and can also be used as a preventative to discourage others from settling in.

25ml (1 fl oz) olive oil
25ml (1 fl oz) neem oil
10–20 drops essential oils
   (choose a mixture from the list left)

Combine the oils and essential oils in a bowl. Massage the mixture over dry hair, brush through and cover with a swimming or shower cap. Leave for at least 4 hours or overnight.

Comb through hair with a fine nit comb to remove any lice and eggs (dead or alive). To wash the oily solution off, apply a liberal amount of shampoo to the oil-soaked hair (without adding water), massage well, rinse and repeat. Repeat the treatment for a few days running if necessary.

RINGWORM
See page 130.

ECZEMA
See page 126.

Benign enlargement of the prostate gland (benign prostatic hyperplasia, or BPH) affects many men from middle age onwards. The prostate gland is a small gland that sits just beneath the bladder and provides fluid for sperm production. If it becomes enlarged it can restrict the flow of urine, causing an increased urge to urinate, dribbling and urine infections. If you suffer from these symptoms, see a medical doctor to rule out any other underlying conditions.

The exact cause of prostate enlargement is unknown, but it has been linked to hormonal changes that occur with ageing. The two main herbs used to treat the prostate are saw palmetto and nettle root, but this condition is best treated under the supervision of a herbalist.

Prostatitis is an acute inflammation of the prostate usually caused by bacteria. The symptoms are similar to cystitis (page 157) and are treated herbally in much the same way.

HERBS *Saw palmetto, nettle root, echinacea, ginseng*

Sadly, there are no magic herbs for reducing hair loss, which is determined by many factors including a genetic predisposition. However, ensuring a balanced diet and plenty of exercise will go far to making sure you optimise the ability to grow healthy hair. You can also use hair and scalp rinses or hair balm to aid healthy scalp and hair, which in turn can help growth. See also page 134.

RECIPES *Herbal hair rinse (page 135); Castor oil hair-conditioning mask (page 137)*

Shaving rash

Men with sensitive skin can suffer from shaving rash, ingrowing hairs and infection of the hair follicles. Ensure you maintain a regular skincare regime using a good-quality, natural cleanser, toner and moisturiser. The aftershave recipe below contains healing and antimicrobial herbs to help soothe the skin and prevent infection and spots after shaving. The herbs below can also be infused and the liquid used as a wash to heal small shaving wounds.

EXTERNAL HERBS *Calendula, thyme, gotu kola, oats*

RECIPES *Wound wash (page 38); Skin-soothing gel (page 44) Aftershave gel (below); Beard oil (opposite); Nourishing skin cream (page 123); Floral face toner (page 131);*

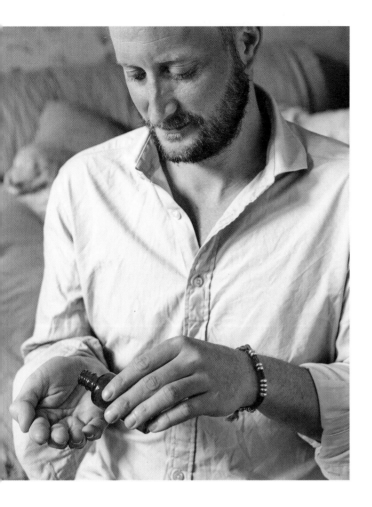

Beard oil

A beard oil to encourage healthy growth, and to soften and scent facial hair.

50ml (2 fl oz) calendula infused jojoba oil
50ml (2 fl oz) rosemary infused castor oil
5 drops lavender essential oil
10 drops rosemary essential oil
10 drops juniper essential oil

Combine the above oils in a 100ml (3 fl oz) pump bottle and shake well to combine. Label and date the bottle.

TO USE Place a little in the palm of the hand and massage well into the beard area.

SHELF LIFE Up to 1 year in a cool, dark place.

Aftershave gel

The antimicrobial oils combined with soothing aloe create a cooling aftershave to help heal cuts and prevent infection.

250ml (9 fl oz) aloe vera gel
1 tablespoon jojoba oil,
   or calendula infused jojoba oil
1 tablespoon witch hazel
1 teaspoon glycerine
5 drops juniper essential oil
5 drops lemon eucalyptus essential oil
5 drops rosemary essential oil

Place the aloe vera in a bowl and gently whisk in the other ingredients one at a time, little by little, until well combined. Store in a jar in a dark, cool dry place. Label and date the jar.

TO USE Smooth a little onto the face after shaving.

SHELF LIFE Up to 3 months in a cool, dark place.

JOCK ITCH/RINGWORM

The crotch area is warm and damp, making it an ideal place for fungal overgrowth, which can cause an irritating itchy skin infection. The fungus that causes this, tinea cruris, is in the same group of fungi that cause athlete's foot and ringworm. Boosting the immune system (page 74), taking bitter and lymphatic skin-clearing herbs and applying topical antifungal preparations are the traditional approaches to treating the underlying problems. Take a few drops of burdock tincture in a little water three times a day. Alongside this, use herbal washes, antifungal herbs and treatments such as the antifungal powder (right) daily.

INTERNAL HERBS *Thyme, sage, oregano, calendula, pau d'arco, echinacea, elderberry, burdock, dandelion, dock*

EXTERNAL HERBS *Thyme, sage, oregano, calendula, tea tree, lavender, eucalyptus, myrrh*

RECIPES *Antimicrobial gel (page 37); Immune tincture (page 80); Anti-fungal powder (right)*

Antifungal powder

Fungi like to live in a warm, damp environment, hence the tendency for infection around the feet and groin area. This drying powder helps to make the environment inhospitable for fungal growth and is boosted with antifungal essential oils, which makes it smell lovely, too.

65g (2¼ oz) cornflour
75g (2½ oz) bentonite clay
½ teaspoon turmeric powder
10 drops lavender essential oil
10 drops thyme essential oil
10 drops eucalyptus essential oil
10 drops oregano essential oil

Place the cornflour and clay in a pestle and mortar or blender and add the essential oils drop by drop. Grind or pulse the oils into the powder until combined. Store in an airtight container.

TO USE Apply to affected area 1–3 times a day.

SHELF LIFE Will keep in an airtight container in a cool, dark place for up to 12 months.

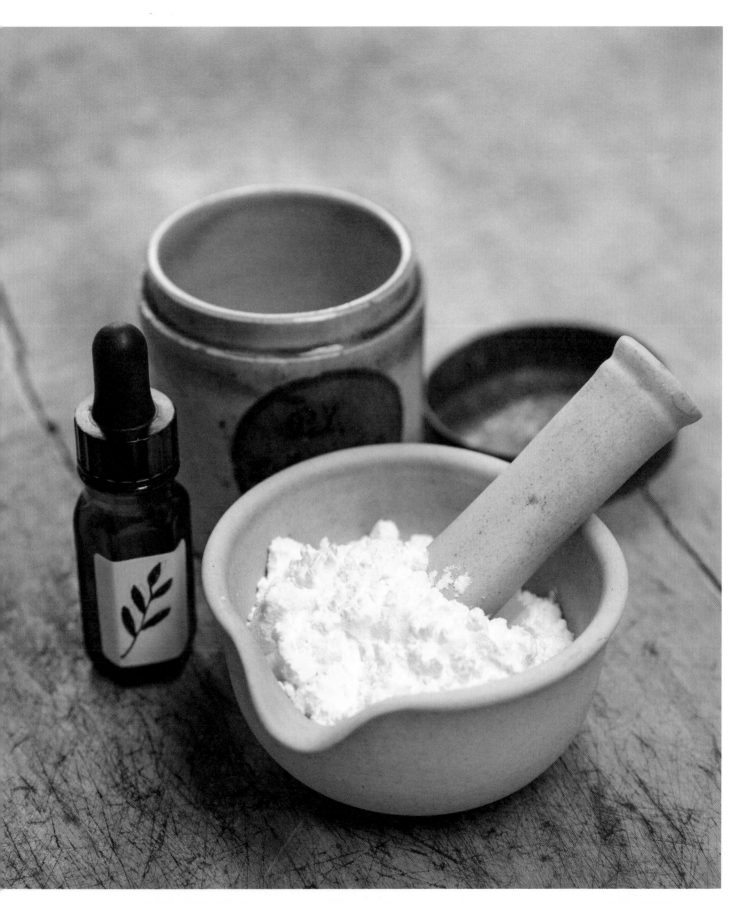

WOMEN'S HEALTH
HEAVY PERIODS

Heavy menstrual bleeding can be a sign of an underlying hormonal imbalance or gynaecological problem, especially if bleeding becomes heavier than usual; it is important to have any sudden changes in the menstrual cycle investigated by a healthcare practitioner. However, some women suffer from heavy periods without an underlying problem. In this case, heavy bleeding is usually caused by a mild hormonal imbalance and/or thicker than average uterine lining.

If you suffer from heavy periods it is important to keep iron and other minerals such as magnesium high in the diet (see Anaemia, page 54). Certain herbs have been used traditionally to 'tone' the uterus, such as raspberry leaf or lady's mantle, which can help to lessen bleeding. These herbs are mineral-rich, too, and the best way to take them is in daily hot or cold, long/overnight infusions (page 12).

INTERNAL HERBS *Raspberry leaf, lady's mantle, yarrow, shepherd's purse, self-heal, calendula*

RECIPES *Nettle soup (page 54); Nettle iron drops (page 56); Womb-tone-tea (right); Ashwagandha, flax & chia seed pudding (page 152); Mineral-rich overnight infusion (page 152); Dark & moody truffles (page 154)*

Womb-tone tea

This tea combines mineral-rich herbs to help counter mineral loss associated with heavy periods. Lady's mantle and raspberry leaf are traditionally used for balancing the female hormones and toning the female reproductive system.

raspberry leaf
lady's mantle
nettle leaf

Mix together equal amounts of each herb (a handful of each should be enough to last a few weeks) and store in an airtight container.

TO USE Add 1–2 teaspoons of the mixed herbs to each cup of boiling water. cover and Infuse for 5–10 minutes or overnight, then strain out the herbs and retain the liquid. Drink 1 cup 1–3 times a day.

SHELF LIFE The dried herb tea will keep in an airtight container in a cool, dark place for up to 2 years.

ANAEMIA

See page 54.

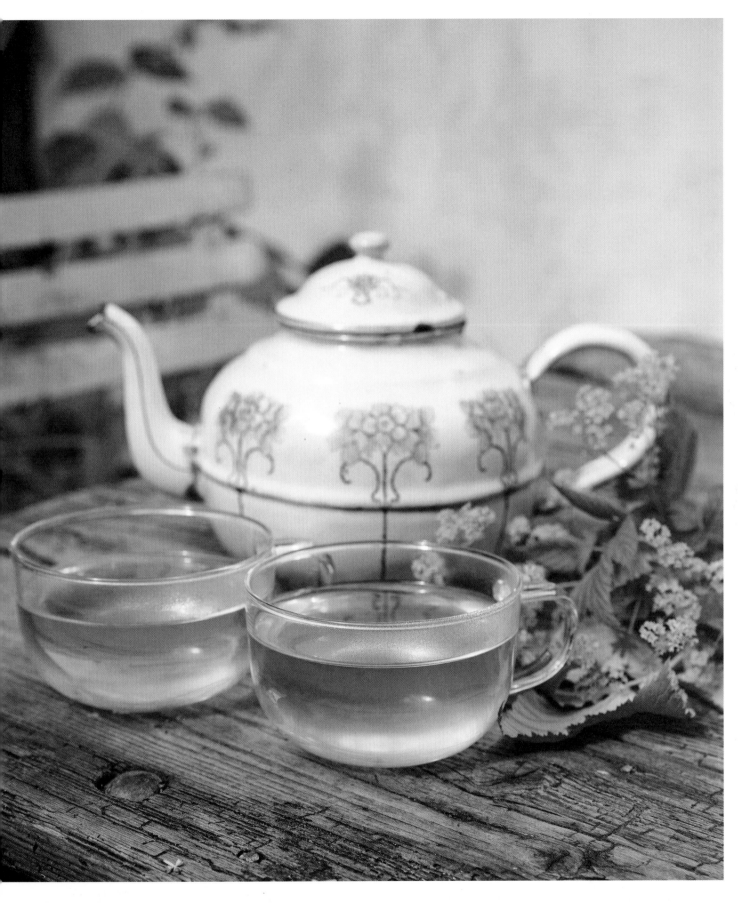

PERIOD PAIN

The pain that many women experience during their period is caused by the uterine muscles cramping down to shed the lining of the womb, and vary in severity from woman to woman. Severe pain, especially if out of the ordinary for you, can be a sign of an underlying gynaecological or hormonal problem and should be checked out by a doctor. Some women experience more pain than others for many reasons, including the shape and position of the uterus, how the uterus contracts, and how blood flow is affected by various naturally occurring pain chemicals in the body.

Taking an omega-3-rich oil such as fish oils or algae supplements in the week before menstruation can help to reduce period pain. Womb-toning herbs can help to strengthen the uterine muscles, reducing inefficient cramping and in turn period pain. Magnesium helps with proper function of muscle contraction; increase it in the diet before and during the first few days of your period, or use supplements. A warming rub massaged on the abdomen and back will help relax muscles.

INTERNAL HERBS *Lady's mantle, cramp bark, meadowsweet, calendula, chamomile, yarrow, ginger, California poppy, juniper*

RECIPES *Chilli & ginger joint rub (page 96); Womb-tone tea (page 148); Cramp drops (right); Dark & moody truffles (page 154)*

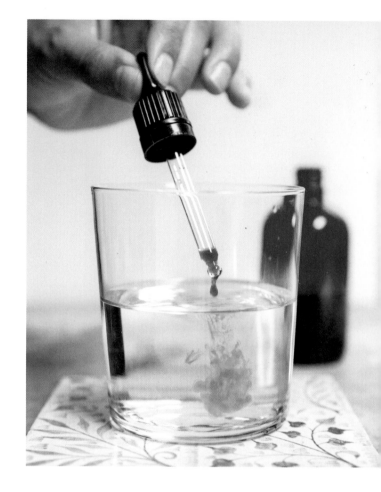

Cramp drops

This tincture mix contains herbs that tighten and tone the womb and help lessen intense cramping. Begin taking it one week before menstruation and during the first few days of menstrual cramps.

50ml (2 fl oz) cramp bark tincture
50ml (2 fl oz) lady's mantle tincture
50ml (2 fl oz) raspberry leaf tincture
5ml (1 teaspoon) ginger tincture

Mix all the tinctures together and pour into a dark glass bottle. Label and date the bottle.

TO USE Take 5ml of the tincture in a little water 3 times a day during the week prior to the period and during menstruation.

SHELF LIFE Up to 2 years in a cool, dark place.

MENOPAUSE

Menopause is the natural cessation of the menstrual cycle, and usually occurs between the ages of 45 and 55 due to a decline in oestrogen levels. While the menopause is a completely natural part of life for all women, the symptoms that accompany it can be uncomfortable. These include: hot flushes, vaginal dryness, low mood, anxiety, forgetfulness, low libido, amongst others. If any of these symptoms are severe or affecting your quality of life, it may be worth seeing a herbalist to get the most effective holistic treatment tailored to individual needs. For mild symptoms, treatment at home can be an effective way to alleviate discomfort.

Herbs containing phytoestrogens (plant-based oestrogen-like compounds) such as red clover can be helpful here; they work by sitting in the same hormone receptors as the body's own oestrogen, meaning that there is more free circulating oestrogen in the body. It is essential to keep calcium and other bone minerals abundant in the diet around the time of the menopause. This is because the reduction in oestrogen in the body can also cause bone density loss (see Osteoporosis, page 103).

Sage tea is a traditional remedy for menopausal hot flushes: drink a cup of the infusion as needed; alternatively, keep a bottle of sage tincture to hand and take 20–40 drops in water when you feel hot flushes coming. If brain fog and anxiety are an issue, try some adaptogenic herbs, such as skullcap and ashwagandha, which are great tonic herbs to use during menopausal emotional ups and downs.

During both perimenopause and menopause, take an omega-3 supplement and/or increase omega-3 in the diet by eating more oily fish, pumpkin seeds, flax and chia seeds. Research has shown that omega-3 can help balance hormones, improve mood, lessen inflammation and improve heart and bone health. The Ashwagandha, flax & chia seed pudding recipe overleaf is packed full of omega-3 and phytoestrogen-rich ingredients. If bleeding occurs a year after periods cease, seek advice from a medical practitioner.

INTERNAL HERBS *Lady's mantle, red clover, sage, flax seed, chia seed, evening primrose oil, borage oil, ashwaganda, nettle leaf, oatstraw*

RECIPES *Nettle iron drops (page 56); Mineral-rich overnight infusion (page 152); Ashwaganda, flax & chia seed pudding (page 152)*

Mineral-rich overnight infusion

Overnight infusions are a great way to release extra mineral content from herbs. This infusion contains mineral-rich nettle, phytoestrogen-rich red clover and lady's mantle (the clue is in the name!) to help support hormonal changes and bone maintenance during the menopause.

lady's mantle
red clover
nettle leaf
oatstraw

Mix together equal amounts of each herb and store in an airtight container, labelled and dated.

TO USE Place 3–4 teaspoons of the mix in a teapot, pour over 600ml (20 fl oz) boiling water, and leave to infuse for a minimum of 4 hours or overnight. If infusing overnight, allow to cool and place in the fridge while infusing. Drink this infusion throughout the day.

SHELF LIFE The dried herb tea will keep in an airtight container in a cool, dark place for up to 2 years.

> **TIP** Make three times the quantity of the pudding and keep it in the fridge in a sealed airtight container for up to three days for three even quicker portions. Alternatively, the dried ingredients can be mixed together in bulk and stored in an airtight container, ready to be mixed with milk and sweetener as needed (this should be stored in the fridge for no more than two weeks as the beneficial oils in flax seed are less stable when ground).

Ashwagandha, flax & chia seed pudding

This easy-to-make overnight pudding contains omega-3 rich flax and chia seeds along with tonic herbs and adaptogenic ashwagandha. It makes the perfect quick breakfast or mid-morning snack for women of all ages.

2 tablespoons golden flax seeds (linseeds)
2 teaspoons chia seeds
3 tablespoons porridge oats
1 teaspoon ground turmeric
½–1 teaspoon ashwagandha powder
½ teaspoon ground cinnamon or vanilla extract
200ml (⅓ pint) organic soya or nut milk
1–2 teaspoons honey or unrefined cane sugar (optional)
a sprinkling of fresh or dried fruits and seeds, to serve
a little fruit syrup or coulis, to serve

Grind the flax seeds using a blender or pestle and mortar, add the chia seeds, oats, turmeric, ashwagandha and cinnamon or vanilla extract, then pour over the milk of your choice. Add the honey or sugar, if using, and stir well.

Leave to sit for a minimum of 1 hour, or (even better) leave it in the fridge overnight. The mixture will become thick and porridge-like. The longer it sits, the stickier it gets, so it may be necessary to add more liquid in the form of plant-based milk or fruit juice if you would like a little more sweetness.

TO USE Top with some nuts, seeds, fresh or dried fruit and fruit syrup or coulis, to serve, and eat once a day for breakfast or mid-morning snack.

SHELF LIFE Keep in the fridge and eat within 3 days.

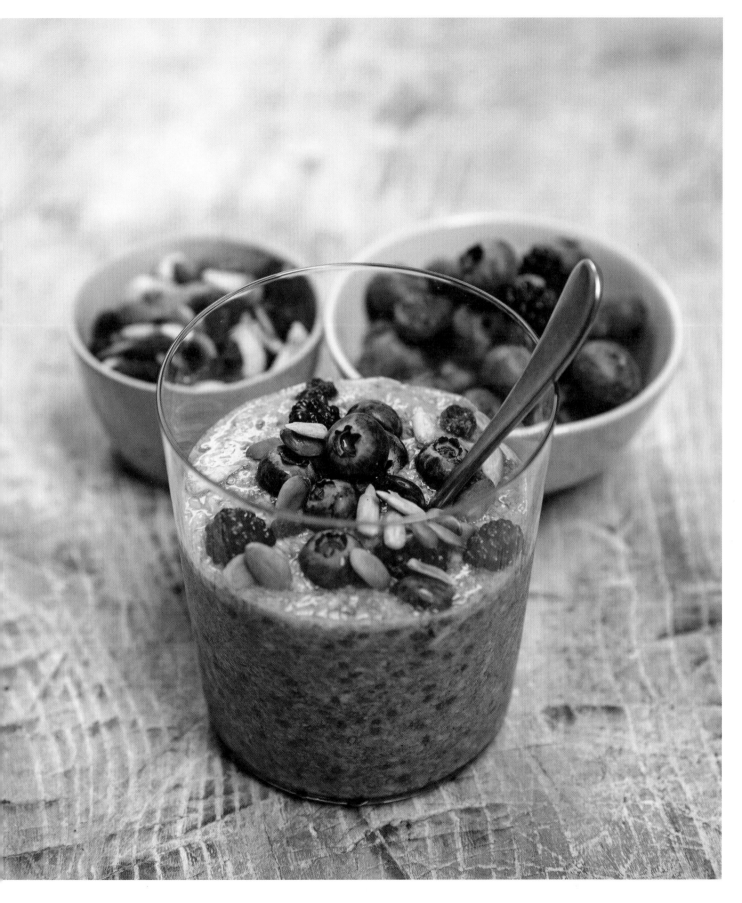

PRE-MENSTRUAL SYNDROME/ PRE-MENSTRUAL TENSION (PMS/PMT)

Women's hormones fluctuate throughout the monthly cycle. Some women experience more symptoms than others, especially in the week running up to and the first few days of the period. Pre-menstrual syndrome can cause uncomfortable physical, psychological and emotional symptoms, including tension, irritability, tiredness, anxiety, aggression, brain fog, skin outbreaks, breast tenderness, clumsiness and low mood to name a few.

Underlying hormonal imbalances could be to blame for those who suffer from PMS/PMT, in which case it can be really helpful to see a holistic health practitioner to get to the bottom of the problem. Simple herbal remedies for balancing hormones can help, too. Herbs such as lady's mantle and red clover can help to balance the hormones. Vitex agnus castus is a great herb for regulating hormones, however it does have a very specific dose, so is best obtained and used under the advice of a herbalist. Oils high in gamma linoleic acid (GLA) such as evening primrose, borage seed and hemp can help to improve PMS/PMT symptoms, as can vitamin B complex.

INTERNAL HERBS *Lady's mantle, vitex, motherwort, skullcap, chamomile, calendula*

RECIPES *Nettle iron drops (page 56); Womb-tone tea (page 148); Ashwagandha, flax & chia seed pudding (page 152); Dark & moody truffles (right);*

Dark & moody truffles

On the run-up to and during menstruation many women crave chocolate! This is thought to be due to a dip in blood sugar levels and an increased need for certain minerals (cocoa is a nutritionally dense superfood!). Avoid sugar-laden, highly processed chocolate bars and try these delicious and healthy truffles instead. They contain chia seed and evening primrose oil, which are high in hormone-balancing GLA, as well as protein, mineral-rich nettles and whole-fruit sugars so you can satisfy those sugar cravings, guilt-free.

a handful of dried nettle leaves
20g (¾ oz) cocoa powder, plus extra for dusting
20g (¾ oz) chia seeds
20g (¾ oz) flax seeds
175g (6oz) stoned dates
50g (1¾ oz) pumpkin seeds
15ml (½ fl oz) evening primrose oil
chopped nuts (optional), for coating

Place the dried nettle leaves in a high-powered blender or pestle and mortar and blend or grind to a fine powder. Place all the remaining ingredients in the blender and blend to a smooth paste.

Take 1 dessertspoon of the mix at a time and roll into balls, then roll and coat in chopped nuts or cocoa powder.

TO USE Eat 1–3 truffles a day.

SHELF LIFE These truffles will keep in the fridge for up to 2 weeks, or they can be frozen for up to 6 months (defrost before serving).

Calendula pessaries

Pessaries deliver herbs direct to the vagina. These contain antifungal and anti-inflammatory lavender and calendula, perfect for soothing the symptoms of thrush.

50g (1¾ oz) coconut oil
100g (3½ oz) coconut butter
a handful of dried calendula flowers
10 drops lavender essential oil

Infuse the coconut oil and cocoa butter with the calendula flowers in a bain-marie (page 24) for 2–4 hours. Strain out and discard the calendula. Add the lavender essential oil to the liquid, stirring well.

Pour into pessary moulds, or use small, rounded ice-cube trays, and place in the fridge or freezer to set. Once set, wrap the mould in clingfilm to store, or remove the pessaries from the mould and place in an airtight container.

TO USE Insert 1 pessary into the the vagina 1–3 times a day. The oils will begin to melt quickly and coat the inside of the vagina, so wear a small, natural panty liner or a few layers of tissue in your underwear. Using these pessaries cold and straight from the fridge adds an extra cooling effect.

SHELF LIFE Up to 3 months in the fridge, or 1 year in the freezer, in an airtight container.

Cystitis is a painful condition characterised by inflammation of the bladder and urethra, usually from a bacterial infection. Symptoms include burning upon urination, a constant burning pain around the urethra, feeling of fullness and pain in the lower abdomen, strong-smelling dark or cloudy urine, frequent urination and generally feeling unwell. It is less common in men than women as the urethra is shorter in women, meaning that bacteria can enter the bladder more easily. For many women cystitis can be triggered by sex, so emptying the bladder after sexual intercourse can help reduce the risk of infection.

Warm herbal sitz baths (page 163) made with soothing and antibacterial herbs or diluted essential oils such as chamomile, lavender and tea tree can help to lessen pain and inflammation. Drink plenty of diuretic and antimicrobial herb teas at the first sign of a urinary tract infection to 'flush out' the bladder and any bacteria. Some women find unsweetened cranberry juice or cranberry supplements helpful to prevent recurring and acute infections. If there is a fever and/or pain around the kidney area and lower back, seek medical attention as this could be a sign of kidney infection, which is a more serious condition.

INTERNAL HERBS *Cornsilk, dandelion leaf, heather, thyme, plantain, buchu, marshmallow, echinacea, cleavers, celery seed, uva ursi, pau d'arco*

EXTERNAL HERBS *(Bath) Thyme, tea tree, chamomile, lavender*

ESSENTIAL OILS *Tea tree, chamomile, lavender, cypress, juniper*

RECIPES *Calendula pessaries (left); Post-partum healing pads (page 163);*

MOTHER & BABY HEALTH
PREGNANCY

HERBS & PREGNANCY

Gentle but effective herbs to help with unwanted symptoms during pregnancy can be found in the list below. They are best used in infusions. If these do not help, ask a herbalist for further guidance. Use 1 teaspoon per cup of boiling water up to 3 times a day. In the first trimester, seek advice from a herbalist.

CHAMOMILE – heartburn, constipation, indigestion, anxiety, insomnia

GINGER – nausea

LINDEN FLOWER – anxiety, insomnia, colds and flu

LEMON BALM – anxiety, insomnia

NETTLE – anaemia, mineral deficiency

PORRIDGE OATS, CHIA SEEDS, FLAX SEEDS, PSYLLIUM – constipation. A simple porridge or the soaked seeds of chia, flax or psyllium make a 'slippery' bulk laxative to ease constipation

RASPBERRY LEAF – mineral deficiency Raspberry leaf is a traditional herb used to help tone the uterus to aid labour and help the womb return to shape post-labour. Use in the last trimester (last three months) of pregnancy.

HERBS TO AVOID DURING PREGNANCY

There is a long list of herbs that are deemed unsafe for use during pregnancy. Some common ones are listed below, but please contact a qualified medical herbalist before using any herb medicinally while trying to conceive, during pregnancy or while breastfeeding.

Aloe (internal)	Liquorice
Angelica	Mahonia
Ashwagandha	Motherwort
Celery seed	Mugwort
Comfrey	Sage
Devil's claw	Schisandra
Elecampane	Shepherd's purse
Feverfew	St John's wort
Ginseng	Thyme
Gotu kola	Turmeric
Juniper	Wood betony
Lady's mantle	Yarrow

Also, a number of culinary herbs should not be used in excessive or medicinal quantities during pregnancy, although moderate amounts in food are considered safe.

MORNING SICKNESS

The first trimester (first three months) of pregnancy can result in a spectrum of symptoms, including fatigue and nausea. Ginger is the number one herb for morning sickness. Like all things during pregnancy, don't overdo it with ginger. Just one teaspoon of grated fresh ginger root or ¼–½ teaspoon of dried ginger root powder added to a cup (240ml/9 fl oz) of boiling water is enough to make a tummy-soothing tea to drink a couple of times a day (three cups per day maximum). Gentle bitter herbs such as a simple chamomile tea or a couple of drops of chamomile tincture on the tongue can also help with nausea.

INTERNAL HERBS *Chamomile, ginger*

RECIPES *Nettle soup (page 54); Crystallised ginger & lemon (right); Happy mummy spray (page 164)*

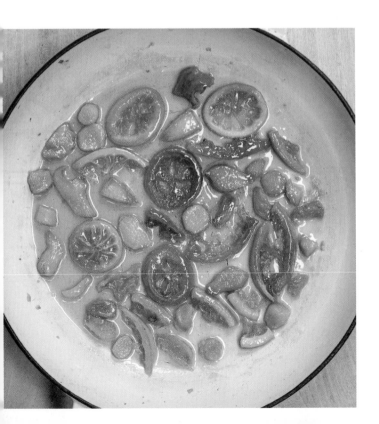

Crystallised ginger & lemon

These can help settle the queasiness and nausea of morning sickness and are helpful for travel sickness, too.

250g (9oz) fresh ginger root, peeled and sliced
   or cubed as required
1–2 unwaxed lemons, sliced
250g (9oz) sugar or 340g (12oz) honey

Place the ginger and lemon slices in a heavy bottomed pan. Keep the lemon slices whole as they crystallise better this way and can be chopped up smaller afterwards. Pour in enough water to cover and bring to the boil over a medium-low heat, then reduce to a gentle simmer. Cook for about 30–40 minutes, topping up with water as necessary, until the pieces are tender, with around 50ml (2 fl oz) of water remaining.

Sprinkle in the sugar or honey, stirring gently to coat the ginger and lemon pieces. Return to a simmer over a gentle heat until a syrup forms and the pieces are glazed and sticky. Place the pieces on a baking-parchment-lined tray to cool. Retain the cooking liquid for another use, such as drizzling over fruit or ice cream or adding to hot water for a sweet ginger and lemon tea.

TO USE Suck or chew 1–2 pieces as needed.

SHELF LIFE Will keep in an airtight container in the fridge for up to 2 months.

STRETCH MARKS

Stretch marks, those silvery lines that signify growth, often appear during adolescent growth spurts, weight gain and particularly during pregnancy. Try the Supple skin balm (right) to moisturise the skin and encourage cell growth while your baby bump is growing.

EXTERNAL HERBS *Gotu kola infused oil (post-pregnancy), calendula, rosehip oil, wheatgrass oil, jojoba oil, shea butter, cocoa butter*

MOISTURISING TIP

When using a balm or mosituriser, apply after getting out of the shower or bath. The oils will soak in easier while your skin is warm and damp, trapping in moisture for an extra skin boost.

Supple skin balm

The rosehip, frankincense and vitamin E oils help nourish and encourage healthy skin, and calendula aids cell regeneration and elasticity.

50g (1¾ oz) cocoa butter
25g (1oz) shea butter
25ml (1 fl oz) rosehip oil
1ml (about 20 drops) vitamin E oil
10 drops frankincense essential oil
10 drops lavender or rose essential oil

Place 3 tablespoons of the calendula flowers with the cocoa and shea butters in a bain-marie (page 24) and infuse over a low heat for up to 2 hours.

Take the mixture off the heat, strain out the herb and add the remaining calendula flowers. Re-infuse for up to 2 hours.

Allow to cool for 5–10 minutes and strain out the herb. Stir in the rosehip oil, essential oils and vitamin E oil and pour the mixture into jars or soft silicone cupcake moulds. Pop into the fridge to cool.

TO USE Rub over the bump, hips, legs and anywhere else that needs moisturising once or twice a day. Avoid the face and genital area.

SHELF LIFE Up to 1 year in an airtight container in a cool, dark place.

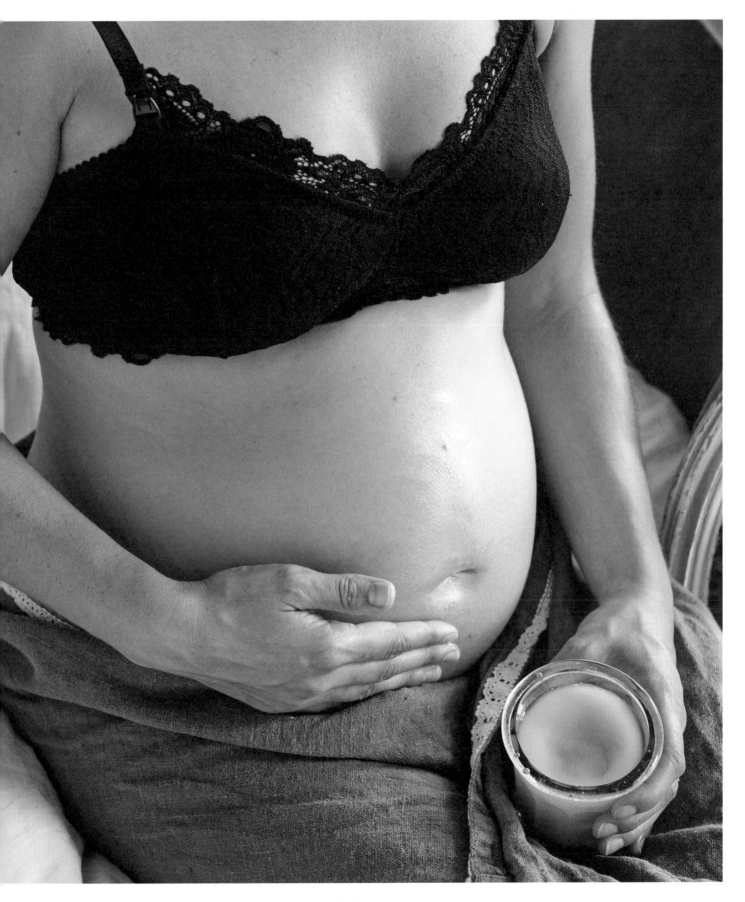

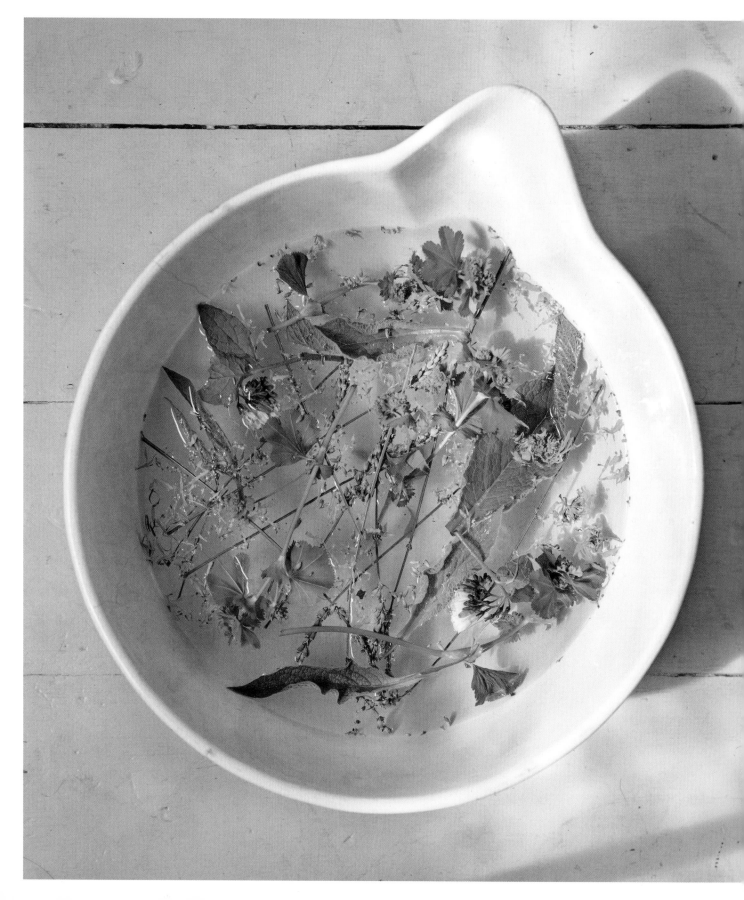

POST-LABOUR HEALING

Post-labour, vulnerary herbs can speed up tissue healing, soothe bruising, help to combat infection, and calm and tone tissues. Use the post-birth sitz bath and the post-partum healing pads in the recipes below to tighten and tone damaged tissues.

Post-birth sitz bath

These herbs are traditionally used for healing and soothing bruised and broken tissues and make an ideal soak for the mother post-labour. Use dried or fresh herbs.

10g (¼ oz) fresh or dried calendula petals
10g (¼ oz) fresh or dried horsetail leaves
10g (¼ oz) fresh or dried lavender flowers
10g (¼ oz) fresh or dried St John's wort
10g (¼ oz) fresh or dried lady's mantle
2 litres (3½ pints) water

Place the herbs in a large pan with the water and cover with a lid. Bring to a boil, then reduce to a gentle simmer for 15 minutes.

Turn off the heat and strain, retaining the liquid, and squeezing out and discarding the herbs. Add the liquid to a sitz bath or regular bath filled to hip height. Ensure the temperature is appropriate.

TO USE Soak in the bath for 30 minutes. Repeat 1–2 times a day.

SHELF LIFE Use immediately.

Post-partum healing pads

These frozen pads use cooling and soothing aloe, astringent, tightening and tissue-healing witch hazel, and antimicrobial lavender and yarrow essential oils for post-partum soreness and tearing.

50ml (2 fl oz) aloe vera gel
50ml (2 fl oz) witch hazel water
5 drops lavender essential oil
5 drops yarrow essential oil

Combine the ingredients in a 100ml (3½ fl oz) spray bottle and shake well. Spray some natural cotton sanitary towels, not to soak but to coat the top layer of the pads. Place a piece of baking parchment between each pad, layered in an airtight container and keep in the freezer.

TO USE Take 1 pad out of the freezer at a time, allow to sit at room temperature for a couple of minutes and use as a normal, post-labour sanitary pad.

SHELF LIFE Keep pads in a sealed airtight container in the freezer for no more than 2 months.

Happy mummy spray

This refreshing spray contains cheery, relaxing herbs to help soothe the senses and reduce nausea. Keep a bottle on you throughout pregnancy and for use afterwards. Alternatively, you can use plain uplifting hydrosols such as rose, lavender, lemon balm or orange flower.

5 drops lavender or geranium essential oil

5 drops lemongrass essential oil

10 drops frankincense essential oil

5–10 drops ginger essential oil (optional for nausea)

100ml (3½ fl oz) water or 100ml (3½ fl oz) rose, orange flower or lemon balm hydrosol

Place the alcohol in a 100ml (3½ fl oz) spray bottle. Add the essential oils to the neat alcohol before the water as this will help them disperse better, rather than just sit on top. Add the water or hydrosol and shake well. Label and date the bottle.

TO USE Shake well before each use and spray the atmosphere around the face and body as needed, then take a deep breath in and out. Do not spray directly onto the face. Not for use on young children or babies.

SHELF LIFE Up to 3 months in a cool, dark place.

Mothers are encouraged to breastfeed to give their babies a good start, but it doesn't always 'come naturally' and it is important for mothers to recognise this and find support from their midwife or women's groups if they struggle. Galactagogue herbs such as fennel and dill are used traditionally in infusions to support breast milk production, especially in cases where little milk is produced. Drink mineral-rich herb teas such as alfalfa, nettle, oatstraw and raspberry leaf in the form of long/overnight infusions (page 12); these nourish Mum, and in turn the baby, and can support energy levels too. Bone or mushroom broths (pages 76 and 78) are also deeply nourishing, helping with swollen breasts during the weaning period. Infusions of sage and/or rosemary are used to help 'dry up' milk once baby is weaned. Large amounts of these herbs should be avoided during the breastfeeding period.

INTERNAL HERBS *Fennel, dill, caraway, calendula, red clover, nettle, alfalfa, oatstraw, raspberry leaf*

RECIPES *Nettle soup (page 54); Nettle & mushroom concentrate powder (page 103); Happy mummy spray (left); Mother's tea (opposite)*

Mother's tea

This infusion uses traditional herbs that encourage milk flow. The aromatic, culinary seeds have been used to reduce colic in babies.

10g (¼ oz) fennel, aniseed, dill, fenugreek or caraway seeds (use one or a mixture)

10g (¼ oz) calendula flowers

10g (¼ oz) red clover flowers

10g (¼ oz) nettle or alfalfa leaves

10g (¼ oz) plantain leaves

Mix all the ingredients together and store in an airtight container.

TO USE Place 1–2 teaspoons of the mix in a pestle and mortar and gently crush to release the aromatic oils in the seeds. Place the crushed herbs into a mesh tea infuser, pour over 1 cup (240ml/9 fl oz) of boiling water, cover with a lid and allow to infuse for 15 minutes. Drink 1–3 cups a day.

SHELF LIFE The dry tea mix will keep in an airtight container in a cool, dark place for up to 1 year.

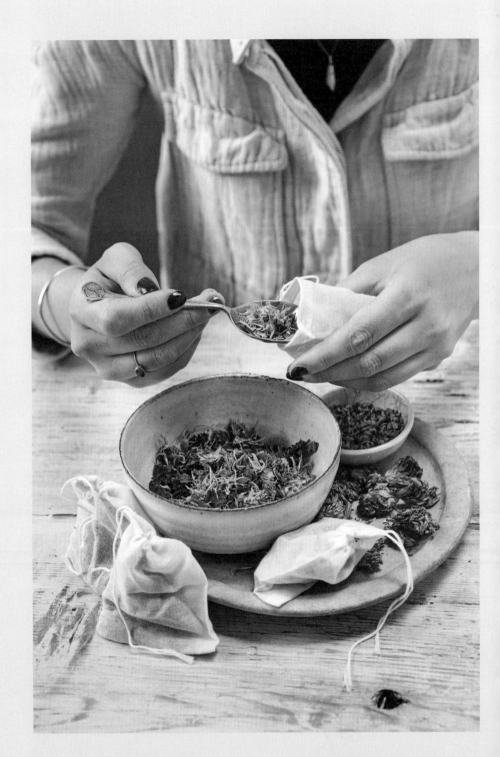

COLIC

MASTITIS

Colic is the name given to long and intense periods of crying in a baby who is otherwise healthy. It tends to affect babies in the first few weeks of life and usually stops when the baby reaches 4–6 months of age. It is thought that colic is caused by indigestion and trapped air, taken into the gut while feeding, causing discomfort. Ensure that the infant is properly latching onto the nipple or bottle teat when feeding to prevent excess air being swallowed with milk; seek advice from a midwife if necessary. If the child is breastfed, herbs can be taken in the form of a tea by the nursing mother and passed through her milk. If bottle feeding, a teaspoon or two of weak herbal infusion can be mixed into the bottle milk from the herbs listed below.

INTERNAL HERBS *Dill, chamomile, fennel*

RECIPES *Mother's tea (page 165); Sleepy time baby bath (opposite); Baby massage oil (page 168)*

Swollen, inflamed and tender breasts caused by a build-up of milk, possibly as a result of infrequent feeds, improper latching/suckling of the baby, or infection. The latter can be associated with flu-like symptoms of high fever, aches and pains and needs to be treated with guidance from a doctor. Herbal infusions and compresses/soaks can help relieve symptoms. Sage and/or rosemary teas can help reduce breast milk production and are antibacterial to help fight infection, but should be used sparingly: use 1 teaspoon per cup of boiling water, and drink a maximum of 3 cups a day for as long as symptoms last. A white or Savoy cabbage leaf cold from the fridge, gently crushed with a rolling pin, can be placed inside the bra and worn for a few hours throughout the day to ease inflammation. Witch hazel water can also be sprayed onto the breasts to cool inflammation. For sore and cracked nipples, try a little calendula infused shea butter to heal and soothe.

INTERNAL HERBS *Sage, rosemary, lady's mantle*

EXTERNAL HERBS *Cabbage, calendula, witch hazel, marshmallow leaf or root, slippery elm powder*

RECIPES *Chapped skin balm (page 109); Breast compress (opposite)*

Breast compress

This gentle herbal soak can help ease pain and fullness of the breasts.

20g (¾oz) fresh or dried calendula flowers
a handful of chopped fresh cabbage
500ml (18 fl oz) just-boiled water

Place the calendula and cabbage in the just-boiled water. Turn off the heat and allow to steep for 1–2 hours or overnight. Strain out the solids and discard.

TO USE Soak clean, soft cloths or flannels in the liquid and place over the breasts to use as a compress; if too painful to touch, use the liquid as a warm soak by resting the breasts in a bowl. This can be used either cool (leave the liquid to cool in the fridge) or warm (gently heat to skin temperature). If using the bowl method, very gently massage the breasts if you find it helps, and express some milk to relieve tension.

SHELF LIFE Use immediately.

CHAPPED NIPPLES

A little calendula infused shea butter or oil can give relief to sore or cracked nipples. Or use the Chapped skin balm (page 109).

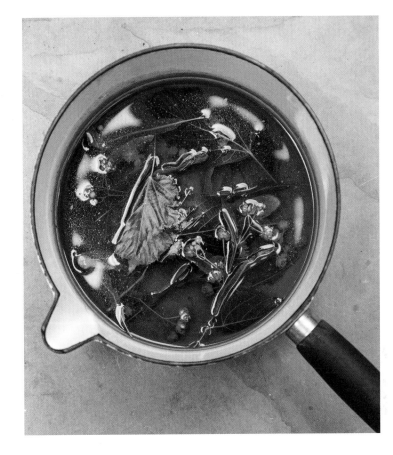

Sleepy-time baby bath

This traditional recipe of linden flowers has been used throughout Europe since time immemorial to soothe excited babies and young children who find it difficult to relax and sleep. Massage with the Baby massage oil (page 168) afterwards for an extra soothing effect, if needed.

1 generous handful of fresh or dried linden flowers
1 litre (1¾ pint) water

Place the linden blossom in a pan and cover with the water. Bring to the boil, then cover and allow to simmer for 10 minutes. Turn off the heat and allow to cool. The liquid should be a deep red to reddish-brown. Strain out and discard the solids, and add the water to a baby bath, ensuring it is an appropriate temperature.

TO USE Bathe baby as normal in the bath.

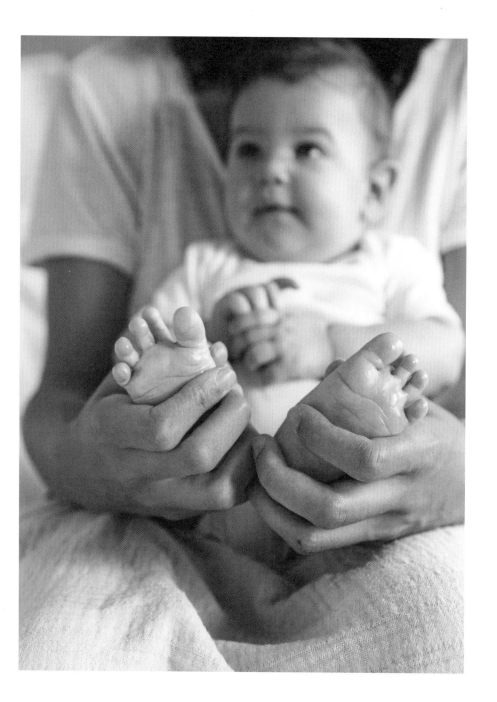

Baby massage oil

A gentle, soothing balm to relax baby, nourish the skin and help the bonding process.

100ml (3½ fl oz) calendula infused
  olive oil
100ml (3½ fl oz) jojoba oil
10ml (2 teaspoons) rosehip seed oil
2.5ml (½ teaspoon) vitamin E oil
  (optional)
10 drops lavender essential oil

Blend all the oils together in a bottle or jar. Label and date the container.

TO USE Pour a little of the oil into the hands, rubbing them together to warm the oil. Massage baby gently all over the body, avoiding the face and genitals.

SHELF LIFE Up to 1 year in a cool, dark place. Discard if it smells rancid.

NAPPY RASH

Babies' bottoms can become chapped or sore when confined in a damp nappy, or they may have particularly sensitive skin. Try to keep the area dry and let the air get to baby bums as much as possible between nappy changes. Calendula is one of the best skin-healing herbs and is gentle enough for babies: a simple calendula balm can help soothe and heal. A traditional bath-time remedy uses porridge oats tied into a soft muslin. The milky mucilage released from the oats is soothing, healing and moisturising, and ideal for babies with nappy rash or eczema.

EXTERNAL HERBS *Calendula, lavender, porridge oats, marshmallow root*

RECIPE *Nappy rash ointment (right)*

Nappy rash ointment

The gentle herbs that make up this ointment help soothe and heal sore and chapped bottoms. To create a nappy rash barrier ointment, add the ingredients in the tip box.

25g (1oz) dried calendula flowers
25g (1oz) dried marshmallow root
200ml (⅓ pint) olive oil
4 teaspoons beeswax
20 drops lavender essential oil (optional)

Infuse the dried herbs in the olive oil using the bain-marie method on page 24. Once infused, place the oil and the beeswax in a heatproof bowl suspended over a pan of gently simmering water until melted and combined.

Pour the mixture into a 200ml (⅓ pint) glass jar. Add the essential oil, if using, and use a warmed knitting needle or plastic chopstick to mix well. Place the lid on and allow to set, then label and date the jar.

TO USE Apply to the nappy area as required after cleaning the bottom at each nappy change.

SHELF LIFE Up to 1 year in a cool, dark place.

NAPPY BARRIER OPTION

Once the infused oil and beexwax have been melted together, briskly whisk 50g (1¾ oz) of arrowroot powder or non-nano zinc powder until the mixture starts to cool and set.

COMMON / SCIENTIFIC NAME CHECKLIST & INDEX

Suppliers of herbs & ingredients

G. BALDWIN & CO.
Herbs, bottles and ingredients
www.baldwins.co.uk
171–173 Walworth Road
London
SE17 1RW
Telephone: (020) 7703 5550
info@baldwins.co.uk
www.baldwins.co.uk

CALEY'S APOTHECARY
Herbs, bottles and ingredients
www.caleysapothecary.co.uk
151–153 Clapham High Street
London
SW4 7SS
Telephone: (020) 3730 4578
info@CaleysApothecary.co.uk
www.caleysapothecary.co.uk/

NAPIERS THE HERBALISTS
Herbs, bottles and ingredients
www.napiers.net
Mail order Dept
31 Townsend Street
Glasgow
G4 0LA
Telephone: 0845 002 1860
advice@napiers.net
www.napiers.net

NEAL'S YARD REMEDIES
Some Neal's Yard Remedy shops supply herbs; phone ahead to see if your local one does
www.nealsyardremedies.com
Telephone: 0845 262 3145
nyrdirect@nealsyardremedies.com
www.nealsyardremedies.com

NATURALLY THINKING
An extensive supplier of bottles, jars, oils, butters, waxes and other key remedy-making ingredients
Telephone: (020) 8689 6489
helpdesk@naturallythinking.eu

BRIXTON WHOLEFOODS
Shop only; supplier of a large range of dried herbs
59 Atlantic Road
Brixton
London
SW9 8PU
Telephone: (020) 7737 2210
www.brixtonwholefoods.com

HYBRID HERBS
Medicinal mushroom and herbal powder suppliers
www.hybridherbs.co.uk
Telephone: (020) 8123 5318

APOTHECA, FAVERSHAM

Herbal shop

14 West St,

Faversham ME13 7JE

01795 227423

www.apothecaclinic.co.uk

HERBACEOUS, WHITSTABLE

Herbal shop

27 Oxford St,

Whitstable,

Kent CT5 1DB

01227 277799

www.herbsandremedies.com

MOUNTAIN ROSE HERBS

Suppliers of organic, sustainable herbs and remedy ingredients

PO Box 50220

Eugene, OR 97405

Telephone: (800) 879-3337 or

(514) 741-7307

support@mountainroseherbs.com

www.mountainroseherbs.com

STARWEST BOTANICALS

Herbs, oils & remedy ingredients

161 Main Ave.

Sacramento, CA, 95838

Telephone: 1-800-800-4372

or (916) 613-8100

www.starwest-botanicals.com

Suppliers of herbal plants

JEKKA'S HERB FARM

Jekka's Herb Farm

Rose Cottage

Shellards Lane

Avon

Bristol

BS35 3SY

Telephone: 01454 418878

POYNTZFIELD HERB NURSERY

Poyntzfield Herb Nursery

Black Isle

By Dingwall IV7 8LX

Ross & Cromarty

Scotland

Telephone: 01381 610352

info@poyntzfieldherbs.co.uk

www.poyntzfieldherbs.co.uk

THE HERB FARM

Peppard Road

Sonning Common

Reading

Berkshire

RG4 9NJ

Telephone: 0118 972 4220

OREGON'S WILD HARVEST

1601 NE Hemlock Ave.

Redmond, OR 97756

Telephone: (800) 316-6869

www.oreganswildharvest.com

The main self-regulatory boards that maintain a list of trained medical herbalists are listed here, but good local herbalists can also be found if you keep your ear to the ground in your local area.

NATIONAL INSTITUTE OF MEDICAL HERBALISTS (NIMH)

www.nimh.org.uk

Telephone: (01392) 426022

info@nimh.org.uk

ASSOCIATION OF MASTER HERBALISTS (AMH)

www.associationofmasterherbalists.co.uk

BRITISH HERBAL MEDICINES ASSOCIATION (BHMA)

www.bhma.info

COLLEGE OF PRACTITIONERS OF PHYTOTHERAPY (CPP)

www.thecpp.uk

THE AMERICAN ASSOCIATION OF NATUROPATHIC PHYSICIANS (AANP)

Telephone: 202-237-8150

www.naturopathic.org

THE AMERICAN HERBALISTS GUILD (AHG)

PO. Box 3076

Asheville, NC 28802-3076

Telephone: 617-520-4372

office@americanherbalistsguild.com

A HERBALIST'S LIBRARY

There are plenty of books on herbs and herbal remedies out there, but we particularly value those listed below, and would recommend them to anyone interested in learning more about herbal medicine and holistic healthcare. This is by no means a complete list, as there are plenty of wonderful books and authors on the subject. We wish you a wonderful herbal journey...

Books

UNDERSTANDING A HOLISTIC APPROACH TO THE BODY

Handmade Apothecary, Kim Walker and Vicky Chown (Kyle Books, 2017)

Holistic Herbal, David Hoffmann (HarperCollins, 1990)

The Complete Herbal Tutor, Anne McIntyre (Octopus Books, 2019)

FORAGING FOR PLANTS

Hedgerow Medicine, Julie Bruton-Seal and Matthew Seal (Merlin Unwin, 2008)

USEFUL 'ENCYCLOPEDIAS'

Neal's Yard Natural Remedies, Susan Curtis, Romy Fraser and Irene Kohler (Neal's Yard Press, 2006)

Bartram's Encyclopedia of Herbal Medicine, Thomas Bartram (Marlowe & Co., 2002).

Collins Botanical Bible, Sonya Patel Ellis, (William Collins, 2018)

REMEDY MAKING AND HERBS

Herbal Remedies, Christopher Hedley and Non Shaw (Parragon, 1996, plus various reprints)

The Herbal Medicine-Maker's Handbook: A Home Manual, James Green (Crossing Press, 2011)

MODERN SCIENTIFIC EVIDENCE

Medical Herbalism, The Science and Practice of Herbal Medicine: Principles and Practices by David Hoffmann (Healing Arts Press, 2003)

Principles and Practice of Phytotherapy, Simon Mills and Kerry Bone (Churchill Livingstone, 2013)

GROWING HERBS

Jekka's Complete Herb Book: In Association with the Royal Horticultural Society, Jekka McVicar (Kyle Books, 2009)

PLANT IDENTIFICATION

Wild Flowers of Britain: Over a Thousand Species by Photographic Identification, Roger Phillips (Pan Books, 1977)

Wild Flowers of Britain and Ireland, Rae Spencer Jones and Sarah Cuttle (Kyle Books, 2018)

Online resources

PLANTS FOR A FUTURE

An online encyclopedia of global edible and medicinal plant uses
www.pfaf.org

MRS GRIEVE'S MODERN HERBAL (1931)

A searchable online version of a wonderful early twentieth-century herbal publication
www.botanical.com

AMERICAN BOTANICAL COUNCIL

Herbal monographs
www.herbalgram.org

EUROPEAN MEDICINES AGENCY

Herbal monographs
www.ema.europa.eu

INDEX

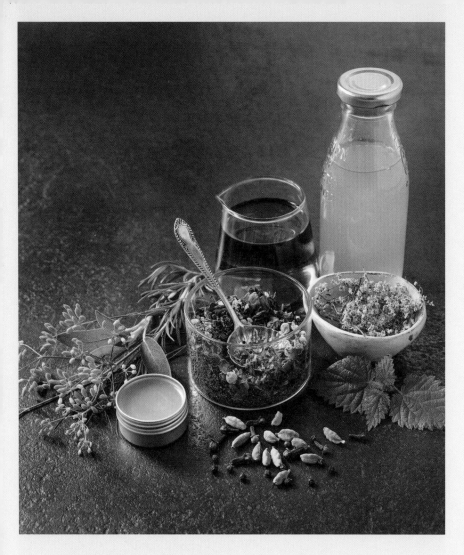

Acknowledgements

To the late, great Chris Hedley (1946–2017), herbalist, teacher (and wizard!). Thank you for sharing with us the wonder and magic of plants.

Our warmest thanks to:
Josie Pearse of Pearse & Black for being a wonderful mentor, agent and friend.

Sophie Allen and Sarah Cuttle for their amazing enthusiasm and vision.

Naomi, Harry Collins, Aisha Turner and baby Elias for their excellent modelling.

Dedications

To Marleymoo, my sidekick and best friend. Vicky

Thanks to my lovely Mum, who bought me my first herbal magazine and let me mess around in the kitchen. Kim x